Dictionary

of Nursing Theory and Research

3rd

Edition

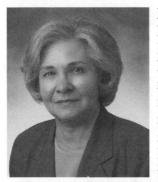

Bethel Ann Powers, RN, PhD, is a Professor of Nursing at the University of Rochester School of Nursing in Rochester, New York. She received a BS degree in nursing from Alderson-Broaddus College in Philippi, West Virginia, and an MS in nursing as well as MA and PhD degrees in anthropology from the University of Rochester. Her published research related to nursing home culture and the care of older adults with dementia includes articles in nursing and interdisciplinary journals as well as a book, *Nursing Home Ethics: Everyday Issues Affecting Residents With Dementia.* Dr. Powers has taught classes on theory and research to baccalaureate, master's, and doctoral nursing students and supervised numerous theses and dissertations. She developed a qualitative research course for doctoral students in nursing that regularly attracts students from other university disciplines. She also is a manuscript reviewer for the *Journal of Nursing Scholarship, Nursing Research,* and *Research in Nursing & Health* as well as other journals in her specialty areas.

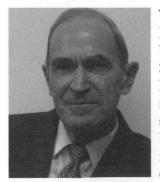

Thomas R. Knapp, EdD, is Professor Emeritus of Education and Nursing at the University of Rochester and The Ohio State University. He received his EdD from Harvard University. His specialty is research methodology (statistics, measurement, design). Dr. Knapp has published several books and articles on reliability and validity and other methodological topics, some of which are now accessible free of charge on his website, http://www.tomswebpage.net. He also served for many years as a referee for research journals in education and nursing.

Bethel Ann Powers, RN, PhD
Thomas R. Knapp, EdD

Dictionary
of Nursing Theory and Research

3rd
Edition

 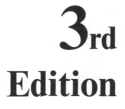

Springer Publishing Company

First edition published by Sage Publications, Inc., 1990
Second edition published by Sage Publications, Inc., 1995

Copyright © 2006 by Springer Publishing Company, Inc.

Springer Publishing Company, Inc.
11 West 42nd Street
New York, NY 10036

Acquisitions Editor: Ruth Chasek
Production Editor: Sara Yoo
Cover design by Mimi Flow

06 07 08 09 10 / 5 4 3 2 1

Library of Congress Cataloging-in-Publication Data

Powers, Bethel Ann, [date]
  Dictionary of nursing theory and research / Bethel Ann Powers, Thomas R. Knapp. — 3rd ed.
     p. ; cm.
  Includes bibliographical references.
  ISBN 0-8261-1774-0 (soft cover)
  1. Nursing—Research–Dictionaries.
  [DNLM: 1. Nursing Theory—Dictionary—English. 2. Nursing Research—Dictionary—English. WY 13 P888d 2005] I. Knapp, Thomas R., [date] II. Title.

RT81.5.P69 2005
610.73'03—dc22

2005011670

Printed in the United States of America by Sheridan Books, Inc.

CONTENTS

FOREWORD

D ialogues about the philosophical underpinnings of the discipline of nursing and the theoretical frameworks that drive the scientific development of evidence for nursing practice have been instrumental in advancing nursing knowledge. However, the progress made has been at times constrained by the lack of clarity of the meaning of the essential concepts and constructs used in describing, explaining, or critically examining the different components of nursing knowledge. In addition, the monumental growth in the knowledge base of the discipline within the last two decades of the twentieth century have also resulted in many new concepts and constructs that were either adopted, adapted, or invented to depict the unique phenomena of nursing practice. Some of these concepts were central, such as "communication" or "problem solving," others were peripheral, such as "paradigm" or "modernism." Yet it is important to integrate into nursing different approaches by which to explain processes for knowledge development. Many of the plethora of concepts used in the discipline of nursing reflect philosophical analyses, theoretical critiques, methodological approaches, and statistical analyses, as well as substantive components of nursing domain and perspective. The well-meaning philosophers, metatheorists, theoreticians, ethicists, and methodologists in nursing have contributed immensely to its progress, to clarifying definitions and meanings of concepts as well as to, at times, obfuscation of its language. Over the years, many, as well, have attempted to enhance understanding of the discipline through shedding clarity and providing direction by which concepts and constructs could be further developed, understood, and utilized in a more consistent way. None have offered more comprehensive analyses than Drs. Bethel Ann Powers and Thomas Knapp in this *Dictionary of Nursing Theory and Research*.

This dictionary is probably the answer to the prayers of graduate students in many corners of the world. It is an urgently and much-needed text that will complement all theory and research books. In this book the authors systematically identify and catalogue most, if not all, the significant concepts used freely (and loosely at times) in discourses and dialogues about the discipline and its progress. While conflicting definitions lead to confusion, in many instances the taken-for-granted meanings lead to even more confusion. The result is often propositions that are ill-founded, dialogues that are less constructive, and conclusions that are less definitive. Critical reviews that could advance the development of substance in the discipline and dialogues that could further the building of the knowledge base turn into squabbles about the meaning of concepts or into defense of one interpretation over another.

This book represents an important milestone in the language of nursing knowledge. It is unusually inclusive of well-supported and comprehensively documented definitions. The authors do not shy away from controversial and oppositional definitions that will enrich the readers' grasp of the concepts, while gently and firmly leading them to more certainty of the best uses. It is well-organized to enhance access, reader-friendly to increase utility, yet scholarly to stimulate thought.

I hope that members of the discipline will use this book well to put to rest many of the semantic arguments that tended to forestall the forward trajectory of the more substantive development of the discipline. This dictionary is a tool that could be used to nurture our passion for substance in nursing.

Afaf I. Meleis, PhD, DrPS (Hon), FAAN
Professor of Nursing and Sociology
Dean and Margaret Bond Simon Chair
School of Nursing
University of Pennsylvania

PREFACE

The *Dictionary of Nursing Theory and Research* provides a compilation of definitions and discussions of terms that are commonly encountered in the nursing literature. In this third edition of our dictionary we have retained and revised most of the terms in the earlier versions and have added many new ones. The new terms are in response to evolutionary changes that have occurred over the intervening years. We have added entries for *evidence-based practice* and *Internet research*. And there are several new terms (such as *intent to treat, number needed to treat*) that are encountered in reports of the results of *clinical trials*. We also have decided to include terms that arise in connection with epidemiological research in nursing. Most of these have to do with the matter of *risk*, but some of them are concerned with the analysis of data collected in a variety of epidemiological contexts, for example, *generalized estimating equations*. Some of the new and revised terms reflect a renewed awareness of concerns about human subjects in consideration of recent federal guidelines. Other new entries reflect increased attention in the nursing literature to the theoretical contexts in which all types of scholarly inquiry are carried out, with terms such as *poststructuralism* and *postmodernism* being used to define various projects and discussion of the epistemological, ontological and theoretical underpinnings of different methodologies becoming increasingly common.

We also have updated our examples and references. There are many fine examples in the nursing literature. We have selected recent articles knowing that they will have aged by the time our manuscript goes to press. This seems like a good place to point out that we think a kind of ageism exists, with regard to publications, which does not serve when it becomes a substitute for judgment. We continue to cite 'classic' and 'solid' contributions whose value we believe is not diminished by time. Also, in our judgment, the articles we cite provide good examples of how the terms and concepts we discuss are used in the literature. We neither claim that they are nor expect them to be free of imperfections and above criticism. All inquiry operates within constraints that are, at times, unavoidable; and the best scholarship invites all sorts of commentary. We encourage you to engage professionally with the examples of your choice in the positive and respectful spirit of which we believe such serious efforts are worthy.

Finally, although we know that nurses have made a wider interdisciplinary impact in terms of publishing venues, we have chosen to draw examples primarily from the literature that shapes the discipline. Since the last edition, we have noticed a greater number of nursing research and specialty journal sources from which to select and have tried to be responsive to this diversity. We also have found more authors and journals from all parts of the world examining topics of concern to nurses in different localities around the globe that are of worldwide importance. Thus, we have tried to reflect what we see as another change in the increasingly international nature of nursing publications.

We do not expect that you will want to read the *Dictionary* from cover to cover. It is a reference source, not a textbook. We also do not expect that you will want to read about every term. Like all dictionaries, it is intended for users who may have very different needs. However, we know that the more often you consult the nursing literature, the more likely it is that you will see an increasing number of the terms we have included in this volume. We have tried to be comprehensive but realize we may have missed items that ought to be included, and included others that might not need to have been. As always, we are grateful to students and colleagues for their many helpful suggestions.

As in past editions, the *Dictionary* includes some statistical terms as basic as *mean* and *standard deviation*, defined briefly for the benefit of the beginning researcher, and others that are more advanced, such as *partial correlation coefficient* and *multicollinearity*, which are discussed in greater detail. We have tried to identify instances where taking note of such terms might help some readers to have a better grasp of the purpose and intent of various research reports. But there are many statistical terms that are not included which may easily be found in a number of excellent statistics textbooks.

We would like to thank individuals who have given us feedback on earlier drafts of this work. Our special thanks go to Ruth Chasek of Springer Publishing and to our colleagues, Mary Dombeck, Jeanne Grace, Sally Norton, Craig Sellers, and Nancy Watson of the University of Rochester School of Nursing. Also, we thank Marilyn Nickerson for editorial support.

As always, we are grateful for the continued support of our families: Richard Powers, Rachel and Jeffrey Wilson, and Helen Knapp, Larry Knapp, Debby Knapp, Katie Knapp-Scheck, and Chuck Scheck.

Explanatory Notes

1. Main entries are in **boldface** type and follow letter by letter in alphabetical order.
2. Cross-references appear at the end of entries in **boldface** type.
3. *Italics* are used to designate terms within entries as well as titles of books and journals.
4. 'Single quotes' are used for idiomatic and conversational in vernacular expressions as well as to distinguish the authors' emphasis on certain words from direct quotes.
5. <u>Underlining</u> occasionally is used for emphasis or for organizing longer entries.
6. An occasional asterisk (*) within an entry indicates a term covered elsewhere in the dictionary, and not cross-referenced, that may be of related interest.
7. Entries are uneven in length. Some are longer because the definitions are more complicated or because sometimes there are disagreements about or different usages of a term. We have tried to point out such occurrences and, as always, encourage readers desiring more in-depth coverage of a topic to consult the cited and recommended background sources.
8. We retain some of our own conventions in cases where there is no consistency in the literature. For example, *fieldwork* is one word, not two; 'ditto' for *fieldnotes*; and some terms, such as *pretest* and *posttest,* are not hyphenated. We also have a special fondness for terms that end in *-ic* and *-ical.* One of us (Knapp, 1992) has even written a poem about their use. Here we choose to be consistently inconsistent, using what 'sounds' best to us in the context in which the word arises. Such are the beauties of living languages! And where better to be so attuned to them than in a dictionary?

Bethel Ann Powers
Thomas R. Knapp

A

Action Research

Action research is applied research that is oriented toward producing innovation and change. Social psychologist Kurt Lewin (1890–1947) coined the term and described the process as a cycle of steps designed for problem solving in social and organizational settings, similar in theory to John Dewey's (1859–1952) notions about learning from experience. Action research can be self-evaluative or autobiographical, involving, for example, examination of one's own caring practices or teaching activities; but more often it is collaborative, emphasizing the role of participants as partners and *stakeholders in studies that are responsive to their interests and concerns. Greenwood and Levin (2000) describe it as *"cogenerative inquiry . . .* in which all participants' contributions are taken seriously. The meanings constructed in the inquiry process lead to social action, or these reflections on action lead to the construction of new meanings" (p. 96). For nursing research examples see Robinson and Street (2004) and Williamson, Webb, and Abelson-Mitchell (2004). Also, the entry on *participatory action research* identifies several forms of action research associated with human rights activism and liberation ideologies.

See Participatory Action Research.

Aesthetic Inquiry

Aesthetic knowledge, which is the focus of this type of inquiry, deals with art and perception of meaning through symbolic representations such as fictional narratives, poetry, drawings, paintings, sculpture, music, films, and photographs. *Human science researchers regularly use the worlds of art and literature as data sources that stimulate reflection, promote insights, and facilitate writing about lived experience (Munhall, 1994; van Manen, 1990). In nursing, Benner's use of phenomenological hermeneutic approaches to explore the art of nursing (i.e., the intuitive aspects of skill acquisition and clinical judgment that are derived from experience) has contributed to the development of aesthetic inquiry (see Benner 1983, 1984; Benner & Tanner, 1987; Benner & Wrubel, 1989). J. Watson (1985, 1994) has used poetizing about caring and nursing as a form of *aesthetic inquiry*. Also, Chinn's (1994) work has advanced aesthetic inquiry in nursing through a blending of practices from hermeneutic traditions (human science) and art criticism (humanities). Features of her method of aesthetic experiential criticism include (a) immersion in self-reflective processes that produce descriptions of the art/act of nursing, (b) use of personal journaling as a tool for self-reflection and criticism, and (c) documentation of individual criticism that "develops from reflections on narrative vignettes, photographs, or other material representations shared in discussion, or from direct observation of a nurse's practice" (p. 34).

See **Aesthetic Knowing, Lifeworld/Lived Experience,** and **Hermeneutics.**

Aesthetic Knowing

Aesthetic knowing (Carper, 1978) is an ability to sense and comprehend the meanings that an art form conveys, to appreciate the uniqueness and skills of the artist, and to develop a *feel* for art or aesthetic expression (Chinn, Maeve, & Bostick, 1997).

> In order to be skilled at the art of nursing [for example], the practitioner, the nurse artist, develops not only the ability to practice the art of nursing, but also develops aesthetic knowing or connoisseurship [Eisner, 1985]—a keenly trained 'eye' and 'ear' and 'feel' for the art (p. 85).

Nurses may call upon their creative, imaginative abilities to share perceptions of what is deeply meaningful about their practice experiences with others. See, for example, Leight's (2002) discussion of storytelling as a useful strategy to inform aesthetic knowing in women's health nursing and Kidd and Tusaie's (2004) analysis of the use of poetry to understand the experience of student nurses in mental health clinics.

See **Patterns of Knowing** and **Aesthetic Inquiry.**

Alternative Hypothesis

An *alternative hypothesis* is a hypothesis that is pitted against the null hypothesis. It often emerges from theory and is the hypothesis that the investigator usually believes to be true prior to carrying out the research. An alternative hypothesis is 'accepted' when the null hypothesis is rejected, or rejected when the null hypothesis is 'accepted.' (The word *accepted* is set off in quotation marks because it does not mean that the null hypothesis has been proven to be true. It means only that the evidence against it is not sufficiently strong.)

Alternative hypotheses can be specific or nonspecific, and directional (with respect to the null hypothesis) or nondirectional. In contrast, null hypotheses, to be directly testable, must be specific.

Example: The null hypothesis that there is no relationship between age and pulse rate has several alternatives, including (a) there is an inverse relationship of –.50 (specific, directional); (b) the absolute value of the relationship is .50 (specific, nondirectional); (c) there is an inverse relationship (nonspecific, directional); and (d) there is a relationship (nonspecific, nondirectional). These illustrate most of the alternatives to the null hypothesis of no relationship that might be of prior interest.

Analysis of Covariance

The *analysis of covariance* (ANCOVA) is a statistical procedure for testing the significance of the difference among 'adjusted' sample means. The means are adjusted to take into account the difference among the corresponding means on an antecedent variable (usually a 'pretest' of some sort) and the degree of correlation between that variable and the variable of principal interest. The investigator attempts to determine if the magnitude of the difference among the means is over and above what would be predictable from the antecedent variable.

For an example of the use of analysis of covariance, see Long, Ritter, and Gonzalez's (2003) report on a randomized trial of a chronic disease self-management program for Hispanics.

Analysis of Variance

The *analysis of variance* (ANOVA) is a statistical procedure for testing the significance of the difference among (unadjusted) sample means. 'One-way' analysis of variance is used to test the main effect of a single independent variable. Factorial analysis of variance is used to test the main effect of each of two or more independent variables, and their interaction(s). Multivariate analysis of variance (MANOVA) is used when there is more than one dependent variable.

For an example of the use of one-way analysis of variance, see McDonald et al's (2003) article on the effect of diagnosis on nursing care.

Anonymity

Research subjects' *anonymity* is assured only when their identities are not known by anyone, not even the researcher. The most common way that this is accomplished is by the use of an anonymous questionnaire. Anonymity should never be confused with *confidentiality,* which has to do with not revealing the identity of and information about subjects that the researcher has, but has promised not to disclose. Of course, in either case, the object is to assure that research subjects' privacy is preserved.

It should not be assumed that studies involving anonymous data are automatically exempt from ongoing monitoring and oversight by an *Institutional Review Board (IRB). Many do fall into this category, as defined by U.S. federal regulations; but IRB review is necessary to be sure that studies meet the criteria for exemption. For example, by regulation, research involving surveys and questionnaires administered to children cannot be exempt.

See **Confidentiality, Informed Consent/Assent,** and **Permission.**

Antecedent Variable

An *antecedent variable, A,* is a variable that is temporally prior to the independent variable, *X,* in an $X \rightarrow Y$ causal sequence (where *Y* is the dependent variable) and could therefore be playing a causal role equal to or greater than that of *X* itself.

The study of cause-and-effect relationships often includes a search for such variables, that is, precursors of the variable alleged to be the cause (*X*). This can be especially important in health science research where knowledge of what preceded *X* could lead to the possibility of control by preventing undesired effects, or by producing or promoting desired effects.

Example: In attempting to determine whether or not stress (*X*) causes depression (*Y*), an investigator may discover that it is social support (*A*)—actually lack of social support—that leads to stress, which in turn leads to depression. Therefore, social support has an indirect effect on depression 'through' stress.

Anti-Realism

Anti-realism, in philosophy of science, is in opposition to realist assumptions that 'real' reality is apprehensible through sense (e.g., visual, auditory, tactile, gustatory) experience. It argues that some entities (e.g., genes, atoms, electrons) that may be 'unobservable' to the human senses are 'real' and knowable objects. See Okasha (2002) for an overview of this debate and Hildebrand (2002) for a neopragmatist response to it.

See **Realism.**

Archival Research

Archival research is integral to some types of investigations involving the use of archives. For example, historians and biographers do archival research. *Archives* are places where public records or historical documents are preserved. Persons in charge of archives are called *archivists.*

Government buildings, museums, and libraries typically house archives. Additionally, the storage and rapid retrieval capacities of computers have facilitated an increasing number of database archives in all of the sciences. Individual researchers also may create their own archives, or data files.

Arm

The number of treatments in a randomized clinical trial is occasionally referred to as the number of *'arms.'* The traditional study with one experimental group and one control group has two 'arms.'

See **Clinical Trial.**

Artifact

In quantitative research, *artifact* is an artificial result that is not a characteristic of the study phenomenon, but instead is produced by instruments or measurement procedures used in the research. The *Hawthorne effect is an example of artifact, as well as *ceiling effect and *halo effect in evaluation research. Artifact can be discovered and/or avoided by multiple independent measures or the use of randomly assigned experimental and control groups.

Artifacts

Artifacts constitute the physical evidence of material culture. They can be anything produced by humans from any point in the history of human society, such as written documents, records, and photographs; personal items, such as clothing and jewelry; or products, such as art, tools, and utensils. The study of material culture is of interest to many disciplines in history, the arts, and the social sciences. In the health sciences, Dombeck, Markakis, Brachman, Dalal, and Olsan's (2003) ethnographic interpretation of the correspondence of Dr. George Engel, the formulator of the Biopsychosocial Model, is an excellent example of the use of artifacts in research and of the usefulness of these letters (from former medical students, residents, and fellows at the University of Rochester to their mentor) in advancing knowledge and understanding of the meaning of this theoretical and conceptual framework to clinical practitioners committed to the approach. (Engel's seminal paper on the Biopsychosocial Model was published in *Science* in 1977. See Engel sidebar in *JAMA*, 2000; 288:2857.)

Assay

In nursing 'bench' research (basic physiological research), an *assay* is a procedure for measuring some quantity, for example, the concentration of cotinine in the urine.

Workman and Livingston (1993) give an example of research that was designed to test the sensitivity (in the precision sense) of an assay for mutagenicity.

Assumption

An *assumption* is a notion that is taken to be true. Some assumptions are consistent with particular views of the world and of reality. For example, in their examination of different underlying philosophies of science and scientific method, Lincoln and Guba (1985) contrast positivist (P) and naturalist (N) assumptions about the nature of reality (ontology) and the relationship of the knower to the known (epistemology):

1. The nature of reality
   P—reality is single, tangible, and fragmentable
   N—realities are multiple, constructed, and holistic
2. The relationship of the knower to the known
   P—Knower and known are independent, a dualism
   N—Knower and known are interactive, inseparable (p. 37)

Assumptions of this sort are used to support different approaches to theorizing and to conducting research. Although they may not be susceptible to being tested empirically, they can be argued philosophically.

Other assumptions are made on the basis of tentative support through previous research. For example, in research on the perception of risk for coronary heart disease in women undergoing coronary angiography, King et al. (2002) assumed that women are less likely than men to receive counseling about reduction of risk factors during routine health care visits. That assumption was based on multiple research study findings.

Assumptions may be based on accepted knowledge or personal beliefs and values. (For example, Zauszniewski and Suresky, 2003, p. 4, assumed that practicing psychiatric nurses are more likely to read the specialty journals they surveyed than other specifically research-oriented journals.) They may be identified and stated in the written work of theorists and researchers *(explicit assumptions),* but many *(implicit assumptions)* are not. It then becomes the responsibility of the reader to discover or infer what an author's assumptions may be on the basis of other written statements. For example, Fawcett (2000) identifies assumptions (described as *fundamental values* and *beliefs*) in her evaluations of the conceptual models of nurse theorists Johnson, King, Levine, Neuman, Orem, Rogers, and Roy. Underlying assumptions are associated with philosophical claims, which need to be made explicit in order to understand the particular view of the discipline that each model portrays.

Another type of assumption is associated with methodology. For example, in the 'pooled' t test for independent sample means there are the assumptions of normality and homogeneity of variance. Assumptions may also be made about the reliability and validity of study instruments, about the ability of study subjects to understand their roles in the research and to respond appropriately, and about accuracy in data collecting and analysis procedures.

Attenuation

Attenuation is a word that means reduction. In nursing research the term is usually associated with instrument reliability. The correlation between two measures is occasionally 'corrected' for the attenuation that is attributable to any unreliability that might be present in either or both measures.

See **Reliability.**

Attrition

Attrition is the loss of subjects from a study while it is still in progress. In true experimental designs, loss of too many subjects can jeopardize the outcome by altering the comparability of the groups. Consequently, in designing the study, determinations of sample size need to take attrition into account.

Audit Trail

In qualitative research, *audit trails* are created by careful documentation of the research process and sufficient evidence to make it possible for interested others to understand how researchers reached their conclusions. This auditing technique to facilitate validation of research was developed by Halpern (1983) and reported by Lincoln and Guba (1985, pp. 319–320). Six categories of documentation are suggested: (a) raw data—audiotapes, videotapes, *fieldnotes, and other documents and records; (b) data reduction and analysis products—write-ups and summaries of fieldnotes and analytic notes; (c) data reconstruction and synthesis products—categories, themes, interpretations, and conclusions; (d) process notes—notes on methods, design, and rigor; (e) materials related to intentions and dispositions—proposal and personal notes; and (f) instrument development information—data collection schedules, interview and observation formats, and surveys. See Rodgers and Cowles (1993) for further discussion of the types of data that contribute to credible investigations and strategies for record keeping and *data management in qualitative research. See also Koch (1994) for an illustration of the use of an audit trail/decision trail in nursing research.

See **Reliability** and **Trustworthiness Criteria.**

Authenticity Criteria

Authenticity criteria by which to judge the soundness, rigor, and 'validity' of qualitative research were developed by Guba and Lincoln (1989) as an extension of earlier published work relating to the more methodologically oriented *trustworthiness criteria*. The authenticity criteria relate to qualitative projects that are guided by the *epistemology of *constructivism (Schwandt, 2000). These criteria include evidence of: (a) <u>fairness</u>, inclusive representation of the different ways in which informants make sense of experiences (i.e., their 'constructions'); (b) <u>ontological authenticity</u>, enhanced insights and enlarged awareness of individuals' personal constructions; (c) <u>educative authenticity</u>, increased understanding/appreciation of these constructions by others; (d) <u>catalytic authenticity</u>, ability of the research to stimulate action/change; and (e) <u>tactical authenticity</u>, empowerment of individuals to take some form of social or political action.

See **Trustworthiness Criteria.**

Axial Coding

In Strauss and Corbin's (1990) approach to grounded theory, *axial coding* involves the use of an analytic tool called the conditional matrix—a coding paradigm with predetermined subcategories (causal conditions, strategies, context, intervening conditions, and consequences) that may pertain to any given phenomenon. Its purpose is to help researchers to be "theoretically sensitive to the range of conditions . . . [and] potential consequences that result from action/interaction [and] to systematically relate conditions, actions/interaction, and consequences to a phenomenon" (p. 161). Axial coding procedures take place when *categories are well developed. They involve putting the data that have been broken down into the categories back together in various ways to determine their most relevant properties, dimensions, and relationships to one another and to identify patterns—i.e., "repeated relationships between properties and dimensions of categories" (Strauss & Corbin, p. 130).

See **Grounded Theory.**

Axiom

An *axiom* is a proposition that, in epistemology, is presumed to be true or self-evident. Axioms provide a basis from which other truths may be deductively inferred (i.e., theory development through *axiomatic reasoning*). In mathematics, axioms are not self-evident truths. They are introductory premises in formal logical arguments that lead to concluding statements called theorems.

See **Theory, Premise,** and **Theorem.**

B

Baseline

A *baseline* constitutes the measurement of variables or description of a phenomenon prior to implementation of the study conditions, such as intervention, measurement of the effects of other variables, or evaluation of a program or individual performance. For example, in a pretest-posttest approach, the pretest establishes the baseline.

Basic Social Process (BSP)/Core Category

In grounded theory, a *basic social process* (BSP) or core category (that is central to understanding all other data categories) is a theoretical summarization of a pattern that people experience in some life situation (living with a chronic disease; adjusting to a new situation; coping with loss). Generally, it consists of stages and occurs regardless of the variety of conditions under which it takes place and ways in which people go through it.

See **Grounded Theory.**

Best Evidence

In evidence-based practice the term *best evidence* has two meanings. The first is a general meaning referring to the most trustworthy of the results of several studies on the same topic. (What constitutes the best evidence depends upon the research question that has been addressed, and will therefore not necessarily be evidence associated with randomized clinical trials.) General criteria for evaluating best research evidence in response to a particular clinical question include the (a) quantity, (b) quality (clinical relevance and methodological soundness), and (c) consistency of evidence on the topic. The second meaning is a specific meaning associated with an available database that goes by the name of Best Evidence and is available on the Internet at www.acponline.com.

See **Evidence-Based Practice.**

Bias

Although used in a variety of contexts in theory and research (Last's, 1995, dictionary of epidemiology contains 28 entries involving the term), *bias* is often associated with some systematic, nonrandom, usually undesirable phenomenon. However, there are differences in the ways that quantitative and qualitative researchers understand and deal with bias. In <u>quantitative research</u>, researchers are said to be biased if they are not objective when pursuing their research. A sample is said to be biased if it is not representative of the population about which inferences are to be made. A test is said to be biased if it is unduly difficult for one or more segments of some population. Even a statistic is said to be biased if it systematically underestimates or overestimates some parameter for which it is an estimate.

Techniques for eliminating, controlling, or reducing bias permeate the scientific literature. The use of random samples rather than convenience samples and the random assignment of subjects to treatments in true experiments are just two of the many ways that investigators can control their conscious or unconscious biases. Using test items that are answered correctly by equal percentages of males and females can eliminate sex bias in psychological measurement. Dividing the sum of the squared deviations from the sample mean by one less than the number of observations, rather than by the actual number of observations, produces an unbiased estimate of the population variance.

Example: In constructing a test of attitudes toward abortion, one might be advised to select an equal number of statements from 'pro-choice' and from 'right-to-life' pronouncements as the basis for the test items, to minimize any bias for or against abortion that the investigator might happen to have.

In <u>qualitative research</u>, *bias* has a more neutral connotation (see the entry for subjective/subjectivity). If the term *bias* is used, most often it would be by way of explaining about the procedures qualitative researchers use to account for particular points of view in data collection and analysis procedures to those who conceptualize 'bias' as defined above. Often these procedures to ensure accuracy and prevent distortion include: (a) cross-checking informants' stories, (b) drawing on a variety of data sources, (c) critical self-reflection to account for researchers' own perceptions, (d) systematic data collection and analysis of possible effects of researchers' actions/interactions, (e) using purposeful sampling strategies to reduce likelihood of distortion, and (f) constructing an audit trail of careful documentation to establish a means for review of the evidence and the decision-making process on which conclusions are based.

Qualitative researchers argue among themselves about the pros and cons of explaining what they do with terms (like 'bias') that have such specific meanings to quantitative researchers. On the pro side, it can facilitate communication about what is at the heart of the matter, i.e., in this case, mutual concerns about the soundness and rigor of research methods in any kind of research. On the con side, it obscures meaning and thereby perpetuates misconceptions about important differences in research orientations.

Biographical Method

Biographical method is historically rooted in literature, history, and the social sciences and is a broad term for a number of approaches used in the study of a single individual. Creswell (1998) describes some of these as: (a) *classical biography*—reflecting the researcher's use of a traditional research design format (e.g., theoretical orientation, hypotheses and questions, procedural approach, and formal reporting style); (b) *interpretive biography*—reflecting the researcher's involvement in the story through reflections and recollections that are partly autobiographical (e.g., characteristic of some *fieldwork approaches); (c) *autobiography*—life accounts personally written or recorded by the individual him/herself; (d) *life history*—involving the recording of a person's life as told to the researcher by the person him/herself; and (e) *oral history*—involving the gathering of personal accounts and recollections of life events which "may be collected through tape recordings or through written works of individuals who have died or are still living . . . [but] often is limited . . . to accessible people" (p. 233). However, there is blurring of distinctions between these various forms depending on researchers' orientations and working styles. What is characteristic of all these approaches is the need to gather extensive amounts of information (cross-checking for accuracy and completeness), determine how and for what purpose the person's story will be told (relative to the message and the meaning), and situate the story appropriately in historical and cultural context (the larger framework within which the story takes place that serves to explain it). For examples of life history approaches in the nursing literature see Champion, Shain, and Piper (2004), Gramling and Carr (2004), and Montbriand (2004a, 2004b). See also the entry for oral history.

Blocking

Blocking is a combination of matching and random assignment used in the design of experiments. The experimenter first creates a set of matched pairs with respect to some variable of interest (for example, intelligence or income) and then randomly assigns one member of each pair to the experimental group and the other member to the control group.

Blocking is to the sample as stratifying is to the population. One blocks the sample to control for a possibly confounding variable; one stratifies the population before sampling so that the sample will be representative of the population with respect to that variable. Some authors use the term "stratified" to refer to either the population or the sample. It should refer to the population only.

See **Control.**

Blurred Genres

Clifford Geertz (1983a, 1983c) introduced the notion of *blurred genres* to describe an observed dispersion of intellectual perspectives and styles of investigation across disciplinary boundaries that was particularly intense between the social sciences and the humanities. He remarked:

> Whether this is making the social sciences less scientific or humanistic study more so . . . is not altogether clear and perhaps not altogether important (p. 8) . . . The refiguration of social theory represents, or will if it continues, a sea change in our notion not so much of what knowledge is but of what it is we want to know (p. 34).

Denzin and Lincoln (2000) associated *blurred genres* with a period of time (1970–1986) when "qualitative researchers had a full complement of paradigms, methods, and strategies to employ in their research . . . The naturalistic, postpositivist, and constructionist paradigms gained power in this period" (p. 15).

Borrowed/Shared Theory

A *borrowed theory* is theory developed in another discipline that is not adapted to the worldview and practice of nursing. The term has a history in earlier theory debates about the need for unique theory in nursing. However, it is not consistent with the view that knowledge belongs to the scientific community and to society at large, and is not the property of individuals or disciplines. The terminological issue is primarily a matter of context.

> Nursing uses *borrowed theories* originating in other disciplines to describe phenomena belonging to those disciplines, when propositions remain in the context of the borrowed theory. Borrowed theories become *shared theories* when used within a nursing context [i.e., when adapted to a nursing practice perspective] (Meleis, 1997, p. 144).

Chinn and Kramer (1995) depict this fluidity and diversity of theory development processes among professions in terms of overlapping boundary lines that symbolize common interdisciplinary interests involving a free exchange of theory content and processes as well as distinct disciplinary domains whose different aims and purposes require different types of knowledge and understanding (pp. 29–30). (See McEwen & Wills, 2002, for examples of *borrowed theories* used by nurses.)

See **Theory.**

Bracketing

In phenomenology, *bracketing*, also called *epoche*, involves recognizing one's inner state/feelings (introspection) and identifying and holding suspended previously acquired knowledge, beliefs, and opinions about a phenomenon under study. Edmund Husserl (1859–1938), a mathematician and the "father of phenomenology," borrowed the term from mathematics (van Manen, 1990, pp. 175–176). The idea that one is able to bracket, in the Husserlian sense, is not universally accepted. Gadamer and Heidegger, for example, disputed the possibility of bracketing. Others, such as Denzin (1989), describe the notion more in terms of subjecting a phenomenon to serious scrutiny.

See **Phenomenology.**

Broad-Range Theory

Broad-range theory encompasses a wide area of concern in a discipline, covering a number of phenomena that relate to larger wholes, such as a conceptualization of nursing's goal for health promotion and maintenance for all individuals in a society. Other labels that reflect a theory that is broad in scope and deals with multiple phenomena and patterns that make up a larger whole include *macrotheory, holistic theory,* and *grand theory*. Some authors do not make a distinction between *conceptual models and grand theories. However, Fawcett (2000) views them as distinctly different in terms of level of abstraction and how they are used. For example, she identifies Orem's self-care framework, King's general systems framework, and Rogers's science of unitary man as conceptual models of nursing (whose propositions are too abstract to lend themselves to empirical observation and testing). And, she classifies Leininger's theory of culture care diversity and universality, Newman's theory of health as expanding consciousness, and Parse's theory of human becoming as nursing grand theories (theories derived from conceptual models that serve as starting points for *middle-range theory).

See **Theory.**

Buffering Variable

A *buffering variable, B,* is a type of intervening variable that mediates (beneficially) the effect of an independent variable, X, on a dependent variable, Y.

Example: In some theories regarding the effect of stress (X) on depression (Y), social support (B) is said to play a buffering rather than an antecedent role in that the effect of stress is lessened in proportion to the extent of positive social support available to an individual (large network size, density, reciprocity, etc.). This hypothesis is an integral element in the work of Norbeck (1981) and others. Evidence for the stress-buffering effect of social support and coping are discussed by Finney, Mitchell, Cronkhite, and Moos (1984).

See **Antecedent Variable, Intervening Variable,** and **Mediating Variable.**

B

C

Canonical Correlation Analysis

Canonical correlation analysis is a type of multivariate analysis concerned with the relationships between linear composites of two sets of variables. One set typically consists of one or more independent variables and the other set typically consists of one or more dependent variables, but the independent versus dependent distinction is sometimes not relevant.

It has been shown (Knapp, 1978) that canonical correlation analysis subsumes multiple regression analysis, the analysis of variance, and several other traditional analyses.

Wikoff and Miller (1991) give an example of the use of canonical correlation analysis in a longitudinal study of myocardial infarctions.

See **Multivariate Analysis.**

Case-Control Study

A *case-control study* is a retrospective epidemiological study in which subjects who have contracted a particular disease (the 'cases') are compared with similar subjects who did not contract the disease (the 'controls'). The term 'disease' is often used quite liberally to include such things as having an abortion or failure to follow a prescribed regimen of medication.

The article by Polivka and Nickel (1992) discusses the applicability of case-control studies to nursing research and provides an example of such a study.

See **Epidemiological Research.**

Case Study

A *case study* is an investigation of a single subject or a single unit, which could be a small number of individuals who seem to be representative of a larger group or very different from it. The unit of analysis also could be families, organizations, institutions (colleges, factories, hospitals), programs, or events. Creswell (1998) includes the case study in his discussion of five qualitative traditions. However, a case study is not inherently qualitative or quantitative. Stake (2000) explains:

> We could study it analytically or holistically, entirely by repeated measures or hermeneutically, organically or culturally, and by mixed methods—but we concentrate, at least for the time being, on the case . . . As a form of research, case study is defined by interest in individual cases, not by the methods of inquiry used (p. 435).

Case study analysis varies with design. For example, a single-subject study may involve the administration of a treatment or intervention. The experimental design will include recording baseline measures of the dependent variable, introducing the treatment/intervention, subsequent recording of the dependent variable, and comparing findings from baseline and treatment/intervention phases. The analysis is *nomothetic,* that is, focused on finding propositions that may be statistically generalizable from one case to a larger group of which it is thought to be representative or comparing the single case with another known group to identify differences. (See also Roberts and Neuringer's, 1998, discussion of single-subject self-experimentation as a case study approach.)

In other examples of case studies that use qualitative field methods, the analysis is *idiographic,* that is, one that concerns itself with particulars—the unique aspects of persons, things, or events that may be analytically or theoretically generalizable to like individuals or circumstances.

For examples of the use of case study analysis in the nursing literature see Feldman and McDonald (2004), Hurst (2004), Kozuki and Kennedy (2004), and Spear (2004). See also Yin's (2003) *Case Study Research: Design and Methods.*

Categories

In qualitative research, information *categories* (sometimes called dimensions or themes) are created by breaking down data, *coding, and grouping similarly coded data bits. As databases grow, it is important to continuously evaluate categories to determine which should be collapsed into one and which should be discarded. It is easy to develop many categories in a complex database, but too many can be unwieldy. Creswell (1998) says of his research practices:

> Typically, regardless of the size of the database, I do not develop more than 25–30 categories of information, and I find myself working to reduce these to the 5 or 6 that I will use in the end to write my narrative (p. 142).

The term, *category,* also is used by quantitative researchers as synonymous with 'levels' to indicate the various possible values that a *variable can take on.

Causal-Comparative Study

A *causal-comparative study* is a type of correlational research in which two or more groups are compared with one another, either prospectively or retrospectively, to generate hypotheses regarding relationships between nonexperimental variables.

Studies concerned with the association between cigarette smoking and lung cancer are prototypical examples of causal-comparative studies, and most of them are of the retrospective variety.

See Correlational Research.

Causality

Causality (sometimes called causation) is a concept associated with the determination of cause-and-effect relationships between variables. Most authors (e.g., Polit & Beck, 2004) list three conditions for establishing that X is *a cause* of Y (there are additional requirements for demonstrating that X is *the cause* of Y—see Last, 1995, for the distinctions regarding necessary vs. sufficient causality):

1. X must precede Y temporally.
2. There must be a strong relationship between X and Y.
3. If U, V, W, . . . are controlled, the relationship between X and Y still holds, (i.e., it is not a spurious relationship).

The claim of a cause-and-effect relationship is usually an outcome of hypothesis testing associated with experimental research. However, attribution of causality is not necessarily limited by type of research design. Testable hypotheses may be derived from findings resulting from nonexperimental research, and there is no research approach that can actually prove causality. It is also important to appreciate that single examples of research are inadequate to support a suggested causal relationship. Consistent replication of research findings is an important determinant of the seriousness with which claims of causality should be taken.

Example: It is alleged that cigarette smoking (X) causes lung cancer (Y). The first of the three conditions for causality is taken to be satisfied, as it is most unlikely that having lung cancer precedes the smoking of cigarettes. The second condition is also satisfied, as hundreds of scientific studies have established that cigarette smoking and lung cancer are closely associated with one another. Except for some highly controlled animal experiments, however, the third condition remains unsatisfied, as smoking/cancer studies of human beings have not provided sufficient controls to rule out other confounding factors such as air pollution (U) or genetic disposition (V) as cancer-causing factors, rather than cigarette smoking itself.

See Generalizations and Explanation.

Ceiling Effect

Ceiling effect is the phenomenon whereby judges or evaluators score almost everyone, as the term implies, at or near the top of a scale. This makes it impossible to rank-order performance and creates little opportunity for major individual improvement with subsequent performances.

Ceiling effect may be addressed by revisiting instructions for scoring performance and by evaluating the way in which judges perform the evaluations.

There is also an occasional reference in the nursing research literature to a floor effect, whereby there is an excess of scores near the bottom of the scale.

See **Artifact.**

Cell

A *cell* is a portion of a cross-tabulation that contains the frequency associated with a category of one variable in combination with a category of another variable.

See **Cross-Tabulation.**

Chaos Theory

Chaos theory (better understood as *the science of complexity*) is a movement that spread rapidly from its origins in mathematics to many disciplines (physics, biology, chemistry, and economics as well as the social and health sciences). What was common to scientists in these different fields was a desire to discover explanations for the apparent randomness of the behaviors of complex systems. Chaos theory provides a framework for conceptualizing order and pattern in complexity. In mathematics and other fields, the advent of computer science made possible the rapid processing of information that has enabled the discovery of ways to make predictive statements about problems as disparate as atmospheric changes, cellular activity, economic fluctuations, or population growth over time that are dependent on understanding the 'wholeness' of how global systems function. In nursing, Rogers's theory of unitary human beings and Newman's theory of health as expanding consciousness are examples of the influence of this way of thinking. Additionally, Mishel's (1990) conceptualization of the uncertainty in illness theory and Dombeck's (1996) analysis of a counseling case involving spiritual disequilibrium use chaos theory frameworks to explain the effects of these unsettled states on individuals. In each of these authors' discussions there are ideas about how human systems that are far from equilibrium may be progressing, or have the potential to progress, toward a higher level of organization through evolutionary change processes that enable recovery and promote personal growth.

See Prigogine & Stengers (1984) and Waldrop (1992) for more information on chaos theory.

Chi-Square Test

A *chi-square test* is a test of statistical significance usually carried out on cross-tabulated data that summarize the relationship between two nominal variables.

Madigan, Tullai-McGuinness, and Fortinsky (2003) used the chi-square test in their study of the accuracy of the Outcomes and Assessment Information Set (OASIS) instrument.

See **Cross-Tabulation** and **Test of Significance.**

Clinical Trial

The term *'clinical trial'* is a catch-all designation for any experiment in the health-care field that is concerned with some sort of 'treatment' (usually a drug, a vaccine, or a new therapy).

There are four 'phases' for clinical trials. In Phase I trials the treatment is evaluated for safety and side effects. Phase II trials test the treatment for effectiveness and usually involve about 100–300 participants. Phase III trials are usually randomized clinical trials (sometimes called controlled clinical trials) of the relative effectiveness of the treatment (compared to one or more other treatments, one of which may be a placebo) and involve very large numbers (1,000–3,000) of participants across several sites, with each site following the same protocol (research plan). In Phase IV trials the treatment is tested in post-marketing studies for further risks and benefits.

Most research methodologists (e.g., Green, Benedetti, & Crowley, 2002) argue that Phase III trials should always be randomized clinical trials in which chance and chance alone determines what subjects get assigned to what treatments, so that the subjects in the various treatment conditions are comparable at the beginning of the experiment. (They also favor 'two-arm' trials—one treatment group, one control group—rather than 'multi-arm' trials.) Recently, however, the necessity for randomization has been called into question. Sidani, Epstein, and Moritz (2003) and Ward, Scarf Donovan, and Serlin (2003) have provided a thought-provoking 'debate' concerning the pros and cons of randomized clinical trials in nursing.

Clinical trials should be 'double-blinded' (neither the experimenter nor the participant should know whether the participant is getting the treatment or a placebo) but are occasionally only 'single-blinded' (the experimenter knows but the participant does not).

The matter of sample size for clinical trials is explained very clearly by Lachin (1981), Leidy and Weissfeld (1991), Sahai and Khurshid (1996), and Devane, Begley, and Clarke (2004).

McFarlane et al. (2002, 2004) provide a good example of a random-ized clinical trial that tested a nursing intervention designed to increase the number of 'safety-promoting behaviors' practiced by abused women.
See **Experiment.**

Cluster Analysis

Cluster analysis is a type of multivariate analysis that is similar to the better known factor analysis in that it attempts to develop subsets of 'things' that go together, but in cluster analysis the subsets are of objects (usually people) rather than variables.
See **Factor Analysis.**

Cluster Sampling

Cluster sampling is a type of multistage sampling for which the initial stage consists of the selection of groups of subjects rather than individ-ual subjects, with individual subjects subsequently sampled within each cluster.
See **Sampling.**

Coding

Coding is a process of breaking down raw research data into some form in which they can be manipulated, organized, and examined more easily. It may involve assigning numerical symbols to bits of data so that they can be computerized. In quantitative research, a priori coding schemes tend to be developed before data collection begins.

In qualitative research, inductive, context-sensitive coding schemes evolve and are continually examined and refined in an iterative process in concert with data collection. Codes consist of word labels and phrases that attempt to capture or stand for some central idea that the data con-vey to the researcher. However, field researchers often develop more than one coding system for purposes of *data management as well as for an-alytic purposes. Styles tend to be individualized and generally involve numbering, narrative, and, sometimes, color coding schemes. (In *com-puter-assisted research, different programs also present specific coding options and limitations.) Coding occurs in phases and at different levels. Initial coding usually generates 'laundry-lists' of labels that become more refined over time as data are sorted into *categories and some of the cat-egories are collapsed. Descriptive codes identify and make it easier to find different types of data; but they do not suggest what to make of the data. It is analytic codes, gleaned from notes and memos, which begin to draw out and call attention to ideas about meanings and patterns in the data.

In grounded theory, there is a coding sequence. Initial, *open coding* (also called *line-by-line coding*) breaks data down into labeled bits to be sorted into categories. The naming or labeling of categories is enhanced by the use of *in vivo codes* that represent the contents of categories in attention-getting ways. In vivo codes tend to be 'catchy' labels that often make use of participants' actual words and expressions. *Axial coding* involves procedures for manipulating the data by relating codes (that stand for categories and properties of categories) to each other; and *selective coding* involves the identification of a 'storyline' in the data and discovery of a core category, or *basic social process (BSP).

See **Dummy Variable** and **Grounded Theory.**

Coefficient Alpha (Cronbach's Alpha)

Coefficient alpha, also known as *Cronbach's alpha* (the educational psychologist, Lee J. Cronbach, 1951, derived it), is an index of the degree to which a measuring instrument is internally reliable. It indicates how well the items correlate with one another, as the following formula for *standardized* alpha shows:

$$\text{alpha} = \frac{k\bar{r}}{1 + (k - 1)\,\bar{r}}$$

where k is the number of items and $\bar{r}$ is the average correlation between pairs of items.

Coefficient alpha is the average of all possible 'split-half' reliabilities for a k-item instrument. Although it is the most commonly reported indicator of the reliability of an instrument, coefficient alpha is subject to a number of problems. See the article by Knapp (1991) for details.

Example: A 26-item test of nursing aptitude for which the average inter-item correlation is .20 would have a standardized coefficient alpha of $26(.20)/[1+25(.20)]=.87$.

A note of caution: This statistic has nothing at all to do with Type I error or with the intercept for a population regression equation. Unfortunately all three are called 'alpha.'

See **Reliability.**

Cohort

A *cohort* is a group of people who share some demographic event, usually birth. In longitudinal studies one or more cohorts of research subjects are followed across time in order to investigate age-related changes.

The term *cohort effect* is used to refer to the phenomenon whereby a result obtained for a particular cohort may be limited to that cohort and not generalizable.

Example: One of the most interesting and most frequently studied cohorts is the 'baby boom cohort,' which consists of the generation of people born right after World War II, more specifically the birth years from 1946 through 1964.

Computer-Assisted Research

The possibilities for use of computer-assisted data management methods in research are numerous and expanding, with ongoing developments in computer technology and software design. Packages that perform statistical computations have long been available, and more recently, there has been an explosion of computer software for the management and analysis of narrative text.

A computer package is a collection of computer programs that carry out a variety of statistical analyses. Some computer packages are very expensive and require a special site license. The best-known computer statistical packages are the Statistical Analysis System (SAS) and the Statistical Package for the Social Sciences (SPSS). Others that are occasionally mentioned in research reports are BMDP, MINITAB (very popular with statisticians for the teaching of statistics), and SYSTAT. Office spreadsheet programs, such as Microsoft Excel, have increased capabilities to do statistical analyses as well.

Software programs for qualitative researchers provide assistance with descriptive/interpretive and theory-building tasks. Programs for descriptive/interpretive functions permit the user to attach codes to segments of text and will then, at the user's instruction, rapidly retrieve and assemble all of the segments that were coded in a certain way. In addition to these two main functions, enhanced programs perform various special functions, such as searching for multiple codes, searching for a particular sequence of codes, or counting the frequency of the occurrence of codes. Programs designed to support theory building permit development of an indexing or organizing system that can be added to and modified as the researcher thinks about potential relationships within the data. This may include the ability to design and use visual displays and graphics.

While computer-assisted methods streamline data management, it is important to remember that the computer does *not* analyze data. Researchers analyze data. If incorrect data are entered, if the coding is sloppy, or if the logic is faulty, the computer will not 'know.' The computer only follows instructions.

Finally, qualitative researchers, in particular, find that computerization has both advantages and limitations. Richards (1998) explains how the computer's assistance with 'getting close' to the data can be a hindrance in 'gaining distance,' which often is the more critical and difficult task. Therefore, decisions to use (or not to use) qualitative data analysis software (QDAS) as a data management strategy should be clear and well informed. Use of QDAS should not be looked upon as producing more 'valid' results or as an expectation. Weitzman (2000) suggests that making intelligent, individualized qualitative software choices involves asking and answering four key questions, which are:

(1) What kind of computer user am I? (2) Am I choosing for one project or for the next few years? (3) What kind of project(s) and database(s) will I be working on? (4) What kinds of analyses am I planning to do? (p. 810).

Another aspect of computer-assisted research is the growing use of the Internet as a site for recruitment of research subjects and data collection, raising many additional issues. We have included a discussion of *Internet research* under a separate entry.

See **Data Management** and **Internet Research.**

C

Concept

A *concept* is an idea or complex mental image of a phenomenon (object, property, process, or event). Concepts are the major components of theory.

See **Theory.**

Concept Analysis

Concept analysis (a concept development strategy which sometimes alternates in usage with the terms *concept development* and *concept clarification*) is represented by a number of approaches that differ procedurally (e.g., different emphases on the literature review and the use of illustrative cases) as well as in purpose (e.g., concept clarification, developing an operational definition) (Knafl & Deatrick, 2000, pp. 50–51). Many of the approaches in nursing are variations of <u>Wilson's Method</u> (Wilson 1963/1970), an 11-step technique for clarifying thinking and communicating conceptually (Avant, 2000; Meleis, 1997). See Walker and Avant (2005) for a simplified 8-step modification of Wilson's classic concept analysis procedure. See also Ridner (2004) for an application of Walker and Avant's approach to a concept analysis of psychological distress; and see J. Smith and McSherry (2004) for the use of Rodgers's (1989) critique and alternative to Walker and Avant's approach in a concept analysis of spirituality and child development. Rodgers's (2000) *Evolutionary View* takes into account the sociocultural, temporal, and contextual dimensions of a concept.

Another strategy, Schwartz-Barcott and Kim's (2000) *Hybrid Model of Concept Development,* brings theoretical approaches (phase one) together with empirical approaches (phase two-fieldwork) in a final analytic phase (phase three) that produces a synthesis of fieldwork findings, reexamined in light of the initial theoretical focus. For a further application of qualitative research approaches in concept analysis, see Hupcey and Penrod's (2003) use of a template comparison process in an analysis of the concept of trust and Schwartz-Barcott's (2003) commentary on their work. See also Finfgeld's (2004) use of qualitative findings to support analysis of *empowerment* of individuals with enduring mental health problems.

Simultaneous Concept Analysis is a further approach "designed to extend the clarification process originally proposed by Wilson (1963/1970) and introduced to nursing by Walker and Avant (1981) [which] employs consensus group process and validity matrices to develop multiple interrelated concepts simultaneously" (Haase, Leidy, Coward, Britt, & Penn, 2000, p. 210).

Concept Development

Meleis (1997) discusses three major strategies for *concept development*: *concept exploration* (labeling, identifying major components/dimensions, and establishing why development of the concept should be pursued), *concept clarification* (refining existing definitions, considering interrelationships between different elements of the concept, discovering and discussing new relationships to resolve existing conflicts about meaning and definitions), and *concept analysis* (defining relevant attributes/empirical indicators and criteria by which they may be judged to be present in a particular situation). (See Rodgers & Knafl, 2000, for examples of contributions to nursing knowledge and research through the use of concept development techniques.)

See **Concept Analysis.**

Conceptual Model/Conceptual Framework

A *conceptual model* is a set of interrelated concepts that symbolically represents and conveys a mental image of a phenomenon. The terms *conceptual model* and *conceptual framework* often are used in place of one another. In Fawcett's (2000) *structural hierarchy of contemporary nursing knowledge,* conceptual models of nursing are described as abstract frames of reference that address the discipline's *metaparadigm concepts of person, environment, health, and nursing. They are distinguished from theories, which are seen to serve a different purpose, i.e., to address a more limited range of phenomena that may "further develop one aspect of a conceptual model" (grand theory) or "describe, explain or predict concrete and specific phenomena" (middle-range theory; Fawcett, p. 23). However, there is not agreement on whether or not conceptual models/frameworks are distinct from or necessary steps in developing a theory. Thus, some scholars do not distinguish between *conceptual models, frameworks,* and *theories,* choosing to minimize or dismiss differences as primarily semantic while also arguing that how to label one's work is a personal choice and the confusion over the use of different labels for theorists' conceptualizations does not do justice to the importance that should be attached to theory work at any level (Barnum, 1998, p. x; Meleis, 1997, p. 135–139).

See **Model.**

Concurrent Validity

Concurrent validity is a type of criterion-related validity in which the data for the predictor and the data for the criterion are collected at essentially the same point in time.

See **Validity.**

Confidence Interval

A *confidence interval* is a range of values for which the researcher has some specified degree of assurance (usually 95% or 99%) that the interval "covers" an unknown population *parameter.

See **Inferential Statistics** and **Interval Estimation.**

Confidentiality

Confidentiality is associated with the protection of research subjects so that their identities are not revealed or linked with their responses in any way when data are disclosed. Information may need to be linked to study subjects for the researcher; but, in those circumstances, research protocols and *informed consent materials must describe in detail the measures that will be used to ensure data confidentiality. Confidentiality should never be confused with *anonymity,* which also has to do with protecting subjects' identities. However, ensuring anonymity requires that even the researcher cannot link respondents' identities to their responses. This contrasts with matters of *confidentiality* where the researcher has identifying information and promises not to disclose it.

See **Anonymity.**

Confirmability

See **Trustworthiness Criteria.**

Confounding

Confounding occurs when the effects of two or more independent variables on the dependent variable are entangled with one another (whether or not each of those variables is explicitly part of the study design). It is usually undesirable and occasionally unavoidable.

If it cannot be determined whether it was Variable *A* or Variable *B* that had an effect, but only some hopelessly intermingled combination of the two, the results of the research are extremely difficult to interpret. However, confounding is very hard to eliminate, even in well-controlled experiments, because certain treatments come as package deals, so to speak. If Drug A is a pill and Drug B is a liquid, it would be impossible to disassociate the effect of the ingredient from the effect of the form in which the ingredient is delivered.

There are situations, however, in which confounding is deliberately built into the design of the study. When investigating the effects of several independent variables simultaneously, a researcher might intentionally confound two of them, for example, time of day and room location, because there are just too many combinations to test separately or because it is felt unnecessary to isolate the separate effects.

Example: One of the very worst things that could be done when designing a two-treatment, both-sexes study is to assign all of the males to Treatment 1 and all of the females to Treatment 2. If those who received Treatment 1 outperformed those who received Treatment 2, the researcher wouldn't know whether it was a treatment difference or a sex difference (or some combination of the two). The appropriate way to design such a study would be to *randomly* assign *half* of the males to Treatment 1 and the other half to Treatment 2, and to randomly assign half of the females to Treatment 1 and the other half to Treatment 2. This 'blocking on sex' would produce *four* groups rather than two, and the main effect of sex, the main effect of treatment, and the sex-by-treatment interaction could all be tested.

Constant Comparative Method

The *constant comparative method* as described by Glaser and Strauss (1967) and emphasized by Glaser (1978, 1992) as a technique for enhancing theoretical sensitivity is not exclusive to grounded theory; but the concept has been rather closely tied to this qualitative research approach. Glaser and Strauss describe it as an iterative process of constantly monitoring data in order to (a) compare collected data with incoming data being coded into categories to elucidate the properties of *categories; (b) integrate categories and their properties to identify patterns and for manageability; and (c) delimit the theory to clarify the logic, facilitate theoretical *saturation of categories, and ensure parsimony.

See **Grounded Theory.**

Construct

A *construct* is a theoretical dimension that has been or potentially could be operationalized by one or more variables. The terms *concept* and *construct* are often used in place of one another, but some authors make certain distinctions between the two. *Concept* is usually regarded as the more general of the terms. In that case all constructs are concepts, but all concepts are not constructs. *Pain,* for example, is a construct that is also a concept. But *ideal mother* would be regarded by many researchers as a concept but not a construct.

Other authors take the opposite viewpoint regarding the distinction between the two terms. Chinn and Kramer (1995), for example, describe constructs as "the most complex type of concept on the empiric-abstract continuum . . . [including] ideas with a reality base so abstract that it is *constructed* from multiple sources of direct and indirect evidence" (p. 60). Kaplan (1964) classifies concepts on the basis of the extent to which they are observable. His third level is the construct. The first two are the directly observable concept and the indirectly observable concept, and the fourth (and most abstract) level is the theoretical term.

An additional distinction between *construct* (theoretical) and *variable* (operational) is usually necessary. 'Intelligence,' for example, is a construct whereas 'score on the Wechsler Adult Intelligence Scale' is a variable.

In most studies the investigator starts with a construct (which often is an essential component of some theory) and ends up with one or more variables that are alleged to be measures of that construct. But there are also studies that start with the variables and extract the construct. The latter is the approach taken in exploratory factor analysis.

The term *construct* is often used in conjunction with *validity* (see following entry). Construct validity is the kind of validity that is of most interest in theory testing.

Example: Obesity is a construct (it is also a concept). An investigator might theorize about obesity and define it in operational terms such as the thickness of certain skin folds, percent of body fat, body mass index (BMI), and so forth. Alternatively, an investigator might carry out an exploratory factor analysis and have obesity emerge as a 'principal component' of those variables.

See Concept and Variable.

Construct Validity

Construct validity is a type of validity in which the conformity of theoretical expectations to empirical evidence is explored. For example, if a theory postulates that there should be a strong relationship between two instruments and there is actually a weak relationship, then the construct validity of the instruments is said to be poor. In such an eventuality, however, it could be that the theory is "wrong" and the obtained relationship is "right."

See Validity.

Constructivism/Constructionism

Constructivism (constructionism) assumes a subjectivist epistemology (Denzin & Lincoln, 2000) and also represents a particular epistemological stance (Schwandt, 2000) that (in opposition to objectivism) knowledge is not simply 'out there' to be discovered but is 'constructed' or made up (i.e., co-created through the interaction of subject and object/researcher and 'researched') "against a backdrop of shared understandings, practices, language, and [other historical, cultural, ideological, and political aspects of social experience]" (Schwandt, p. 197). Although they are used alternately and in place of one another, Crotty (1998) suggests that the term *constructivism* be used to refer to understanding of the constructionist position and that *constructionism* be used when the focus is on generation and transmission of meaning.

See **Epistemology, Objectivism,** and **Subjectivism.**

Contamination

Contamination is the term used to refer to a weakness of any experiment in which the treatment groups are not kept sufficiently isolated, so that the subjects who are supposed to receive just one of the treatments actually are exposed to part or all of one of the other treatments.

Example: A researcher in nursing education carries out an experiment in a college of nursing in which a random half of student nurses are taught how to give injections using Method A and the other half are taught how to give those same injections using Method B. Since the students attend the same college they have the opportunity to communicate with one another regarding their training, and it is very difficult, if not impossible, for those who are receiving Method A to be completely deprived of the techniques involved in Method B; the experiment is therefore 'contaminated.'

Content Analysis

Content analysis is a general term for a number of different strategies that are used to analyze text. Classic content analysis involves quantification of narrative content according to predetermined categories (Holsti, 1969; Krippendorff, 1980; Rosengren, 1981). The categories are created on the basis of issues or data characteristics of interest to the researcher; and rules for coding and classifying content as belonging to one or another category are stated precisely, to minimize bias resulting from judgments of different coders. Qualitative researchers may use quantitative methods when they want to test field hypotheses; but, more often, in qualitative content analysis, where texts are analyzed in order to understand participants' categories, the coding and classifying of data content are not established a priori. Guidelines and rationales for categorizing qualitative research data develop as the process of data collection and analysis simultaneously unfolds. However, counting elements that fall into certain categories, whether constructed a priori or a posteriori, is quite common. Because there are many ways to perform a content analysis, the logic of the chosen approach as well as the actual procedures will need to be described. See Sharp, Pineros, Hsu, Starks, and Sales (2004) for an example of a qualitative study of barriers and facilitators encountered by participants in intervention studies that used theory-based conceptual content analysis of structured interview data.

Content Validity

Content validity is a type of validity in which expert judgment is brought to bear in determining the extent to which a particular variable properly operationalizes some construct of interest.

See **Validity.**

Contextualism

Contextualism is a theory of interpretation that assumes the need to explain meaning in relation to context. That is, it is the belief that human circumstances, social phenomena, and material artifacts must be understood in relation to the historical period and total cultural framework within which they originally occurred or are currently encountered. Interpretive research traditions emphasize the necessity for this type of contextualization.

Contingency Table

See **Cross-Tabulation.**

Control

Control is a term that has to do with the assessment of causality. Whenever one is seriously interested in the causal relationship between two variables, whether in a true experiment or in a theoretically oriented correlational study, one must account for extraneous variables that might otherwise render any sort of causal interpretation unjustifiable.

There is a wide variety of procedures for accomplishing such control, but they are all of either a *direct* or a *statistical* nature. The simplest form of direct control of a variable is to hold it constant, for example, to control for sex differences by using only males, or only females, in a particular study. This option is often unwise, however, as it restricts the generalizability of the research findings. Other direct methods include 'blocking' on a variable (matching coupled with random assignment to treatment groups) and random assignment alone.

Techniques providing statistical control are the use of change scores, the analysis of covariance, and a variety of other regression methods. Statistical control is always inferior to direct control, as the interpretation must involve the notion '*if* ___ were to be held constant' rather than '*when* ___ is held constant,' but it is the only alternative when direct control is either difficult or impossible, for example, in virtually all nonexperimental studies.

Example: An experimental study of the effectiveness of a new drug relative to an old drug would ordinarily employ direct control, with some variables held constant at the sampling stage and others 'randomized out' in the assignment-to-treatment stage, with or without blocking on something like sex. The 'experimental group' would get the new drug and the 'control group' would get the old drug; at the end of the study the two groups would be compared on the dependent variable(s) of interest, for example, morbidity or mortality. But a nonexperimental study of the relationship between type of drug and morbidity for people who just happened to have been exposed to various drugs would have to rely entirely on statistical control.

Control Group

In an experiment the *control group* is the group that does not receive the 'treatment' (e.g., a new analgesic) that is of particular interest to the researcher. (It must receive *some* kind of treatment, however—e.g., the usual analgesic—since there is no such thing as a 'pure' control group.)
See **Experiment.**

Convenience Sampling

Convenience sampling is the very common type of nonprobability sampling in which the researcher selects any or all available subjects who agree to participate in the study.
Example: College students enrolled in psychology courses provide convenience samples for much of psychological research.
See **Sampling.**

Convergent Validity

Convergent validity is a type of construct validity. If there is a strong relationship between a particular measure and one or more other alleged measures of the same construct, the given measure is said to possess convergent validity.
See **Validity.**

Correlation Coefficient

A *correlation coefficient* is a number that summarizes the direction and strength of the relationship between two variables. The most commonly encountered correlation coefficient is the Pearson product-moment correlation coefficient.
See **Pearson Product-Moment Correlation Coefficient.**

Correlational Research

Correlational research examines the relationships between variables, but unlike experimental or quasi-experimental studies, correlational studies lack active manipulation of the independent variable(s). Therefore, postulation of relationships among study variables in causal terms is risky. Discussion of associations in correlational studies, however, sometimes gives an indication of how likely it is that a cause-and-effect relationship *might* exist.

Questions such as "Does obesity contribute to the incidence of coronary heart disease?" or "Does a person's cultural background affect perception of and response to pain?" are examples where the independent variable is a characteristic of an individual that cannot be manipulated experimentally. Other questions about the effects of various treatments on people often cannot be studied experimentally because of ethical considerations that would be involved in randomly withholding from some clients the treatment of particular interest. There are also instances where random assignment of subjects to experimental and control groups is impractical or beyond the investigator's ability to carry out.

Other advantages cited in the research literature have to do with the capacity of correlational designs to deal with large amounts of data connected with a specific problem area and their strong link to reality in contrast with the artificiality of laboratory experiments.

There are many kinds of correlational research in which the interrelationships of pairs of variables are explored. Causal-comparative studies (either prospective or retrospective) compare two or more groups of subjects on one or more variables to determine whether or not there is a 'case' for causality.

Example: An investigator's report of a strong relationship between type of nursing care and patient satisfaction may suggest that assignment of patients to a primary nurse is likely to result in greater satisfaction with nursing care.

The following diagram may be helpful in clarifying the various types of correlational research:

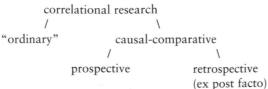

Cost-Benefit Analysis

A *cost-benefit analysis* (sometimes called a *benefit-cost analysis*) is an economic analysis of the expected benefits of a specified intervention relative to the associated costs. The key summary index in a cost-benefit analysis is the ratio of the 'present value' of the anticipated benefits to the 'present value' of the anticipated costs, called (naturally enough) the benefit-to-cost ratio. A ratio greater than 1.00 is regarded as economically feasible and a ratio less than one is regarded as not feasible. Both costs and benefits must be expressed in the same units (usually in dollars).

Cost-Effectiveness Analysis

A *cost-effectiveness analysis* is an economic analysis of the expected benefits of a specified intervention relative to the associated costs, wherein the costs are expressed in monetary units (dollars) but the benefits are not. A typical summary index for an alleged lifesaving intervention would be expressed in terms of dollars per death prevented.

Credibility

See **Trustworthiness Criteria.**

Criterion (Criteria pl.)

A *criterion* is an external standard against which an object (e.g., performance, a report, a research study) may be judged. Evaluative criteria are derived from agreed-upon norms and expectations that are systematically applied to judge or assess the adequacy of something.

Criterion-Related Validity

Criterion-related validity is a type of validity concerned with the relationship between a particular measure and some external 'gold standard,' that is, a measure whose validity has been assumed or previously demonstrated.
See **Validity.**

Critical Action Research

See **Participatory Action Research (PAR).**

Critical Ethnography

Critical ethnography combines an ethnographic research approach with critical inquiry. J. Thomas (1993) described the result as "conventional ethnography with a political purpose" (p. 4). Thus, interpretation of cultural reality is done with the aim of revealing or exposing injustice and giving *voice to marginalized or oppressed individuals or groups.

For examples of its use in the nursing literature see Bent (2003) and Varcoe (2001).
See **Ethnography** and **Critical Theory.**

Critical Hermeneutics

Critical hermeneutics is suspicious of interpretations of experience, assuming that interpretations are prone to unavoidable biases and, thus, "will never be linguistically unproblematic. Typically, within the realm of

C

cultural studies and cultural analysis in general critical hermeneutics has deconstructed sociocultural texts that promote demeaning stereotypes of the disempowered" (Kincheloe & McLaren, 2000, p. 289). Ricoeur (1913–) used the term 'hermeneutics of suspicion' to differentiate critical hermeneutics from other forms of interpretive inquiry. That is, while

> traditional hermeneutics is generally motivated by the aim of restoring lost meaning, and it rests on the interpreter's faith that such meaning can be restored . . . [c]ritical hermeneutic theory emphasizes the need to demystify, to go behind given meanings that are illusory to meanings that actors themselves cannot see (Thompson, 1990, pp. 258–259).

See **Hermeneutics** and **Critical Theory.**

Critical Theory

Critical theory is a term that is linked with distinctive positions often associated with the thinking of specific 'schools' or individuals. Thus, it functions as an 'umbrella' for a variety of approaches to social analysis and critique informed by *structuralism, *poststructuralism, and *deconstruction. It originated in the German tradition of the 'Frankfurt School,' as a neo-Marxist theory of society, a theory of advanced capitalism associated with certain members of the Institute of Social Research established in Frankfurt, Germany, in 1923 by Max Horkheimer, Friedrich Pollock, Theodor Adorno, Herbert Marcuse, and Leo Lowenthal and later advanced by Jugen Habermas. However, contemporary critical theory is more ecumenical and is comprised of many theories and approaches to the study of "competing power interests between groups and individuals within a society . . . [that] often revolve around issues of race, class, gender, and sexuality" (Kincheloe & McLaren, 2000, p.281). (See, for example, the entry on feminist research as well as Ladson-Billings [2000] on critical race theory.) *Critical enlightenment* has been a major theme of critical theory, based on assumptions that individuals are not consciously aware of the *ideologies that oppress them, but that they can be *empowered* through *enlightenment*, and ultimately, *emancipated* by the power of reason that reveals (or *uncovers*) the dynamics of domination and oppression in a particular situation. Another theme is the study of Antonio Gramsci's (1891–1937) notion of *hegemony* that is concerned with the complexity and social psychology of oppression and how its associated ideologies operate to constrain multiple competing interests and maintain consent of the oppressed to the status quo. In the nursing literature see Browne (2000), Clark, Barton, and Brown (2002), Fontana (2004), Fraser and Strang (2004), Kirkham and Anderson (2002), and Procter, Wilcockson, Pearson, and Allgar (2001).

See **Dialectic, Dialogue, Feminist Research,** and **Participatory Action Research (PAR).**

Cronbach's Alpha
See **Coefficient Alpha.**

Crossover Design

A *crossover design,* sometimes called a *counterbalanced design,* is an experimental design in which every subject is exposed to both of two experimental treatments in a balanced fashion. At Time 1 half of the subjects receive Treatment A and the other half receive Treatment B. At Time 2 they 'cross over,' with the first half receiving Treatment B and the second half receiving Treatment A.

Crossover designs are special cases of 'Latin square' designs in which each of k treatments is administered to each of k groups of subjects at k points in time (where k is equal to or greater than 2).

Whitney, Stotts, Goodson, and Janson-Bjerklie (1993) used a crossover design in their study of effects of activity and bed rest on tissue oxygen tension, perfusion, and plasma volume. Also, Sloane et al.'s (2004) randomized controlled trial to evaluate the efficacy of two bathing techniques (person-centered showering and towel bath) for reducing bathing-associated aggression, agitation, and discomfort of nursing home residents with dementia used crossover between two experimental groups.

Cross-Sectional Study

The term *cross-sectional study* is sometimes used in a general sense to classify any study that does not involve a follow-up of the research subjects. For example, a study in which one group of subjects is recruited over a relatively long period of time but is never followed up thereafter could be labeled a cross-sectional study. In its more restrictive technical sense, however, a cross-sectional study is a type of study that involves the comparison of two or more groups (e.g., age groups) at one point in time, as opposed to a longitudinal study that traces a cohort of people across time.

The obvious advantage of a cross-sectional study is economy. One need not wait for 5-year-olds to become 6-year-olds, for single persons to get married, for nonsmokers to become smokers, and so forth. The compensating (and often overriding) disadvantage is that such a study does not lend itself well to developmental, much less causal, interpretations.

Example: A researcher interested in comparing persons of ages 65–75 years with persons of ages greater than 75 years is much more likely to carry out a cross-sectional rather than a longitudinal study of those two age groups. A longitudinal approach to such a study would carry the risk of subject mortality (in both the literal and attritional sense of the word) in addition to being much more expensive in time and effort.

Cross-Tabulation

A *cross-tabulation,* often abbreviated to 'cross-tab,' is a two-way frequency distribution that expresses the bivariate relationship between two nominal or ordinal variables. Contingency table is a synonym for cross-tabulation and is a term preferred by some authors.

In a cross-tabulation, the frequency of occurrence of each combination of categories of the two variables is displayed in an *i*-by-*j* rectangular array, where *i* is the number of rows in the table (and therefore the number of categories for one of the variables) and *j* is the number of columns (the number of categories for the other variable). The 'boxes' of the table that contain the actual frequencies are called cells. The row totals comprise the 'marginal' frequency distribution for the first variable, and the column totals comprise the 'marginal' frequency distribution for the second variable. These are almost always provided, along with the 'grand total' (the sample size), so that the frequency distribution for each variable can be studied as well as the bivariate distribution.

Example: The relationship between sex and smoking behavior for a random sample of 200 people can be determined by displaying in a 2 (male/female)-by-2 (smoke/don't smoke) table the number of male smokers, female smokers, male nonsmokers, and female nonsmokers. The frequencies should also be converted into percentages to facilitate the proper interpretation of that relationship.

Cross-Validation

Cross-validation is a procedure that is sometimes carried out in connection with a regression analysis of the relationship between two variables.

What this usually entails is the splitting of the research sample (ideally randomly) into two parts (ideally equally), developing the appropriate regression equation for predicting Y from X for one half-sample, and comparing the predicted values of Y arising from that regression equation with the actual values of Y for the other half-sample for the same range of X values. The reason for this rather strange and complicated approach to studying the relationship between two variables is to avoid capitalization on the specific idiosyncrasies of a single sample that might produce an unreplicable pattern for a subsequent sample.

'Double' cross-validation is less common but equally feasible in the computer age. It involves the derivation of a regression equation for *each* half-sample and the comparison of the predicted values of Y arising from the equation for one half-sample with the actual values of Y for the other half-sample.

Example: The relationship between height and weight for a sample of 200 adult women might be studied by dividing the sample into two halves of 100 women each, regressing weight on height for one of the

C

35

two half-samples, and comparing predicted weights with actual weights in the other half-sample to see how well the relationship determined in the first half-sample 'holds up' under cross-validation.

Culture

There are many definitions of *culture* but no one standard or commonly accepted definition. Central to many definitions are notions of culture as (a) shared knowledge and customary patterns of behavior, (b) associated with groups of people who interact within a distinct social system or a subsystem of a larger society, (c) cumulative and symbolic in nature, and (d) transmitted from generation to generation. The culture concept, in a classic sense, may be used to direct attention to a social group's or a community's total way of life—its language, customs, religious and social systems, and material artifacts.

In another sense, it refers to values, beliefs, and shared meanings that are explicitly and implicitly conveyed by members of the culture in defined social situations. The purpose of ethnography is interpretation of social and behavior patterns in cultural context. For example, see B. A. Powers (2003a) for a cultural description of nursing home life that is the basis for an interpretation of everyday ethical issues affecting residents with dementia.

See **Ethnography.**

D

Data (Datum sing.)

Data <u>are</u> all of the pieces of information that are collected during a research study. The term *data* is plural, as its use in the preceding sentence suggests; *datum* is the singular form.

Data and Safety Monitoring (DSM)

Data and safety monitoring (DSM) plans are written descriptions of procedures in place for monitoring clinical trials and intervention studies in order to ensure study subject safety and reassessment of risk benefit ratios throughout the study. They are required of U.S. National Institutes of Health (NIH) grantees in addition to *Institutional Review Board (IRB) approval/reapproval requirements. At minimum, DSM plans must include a description of the responsibilities of the Safety Monitor, reporting mechanisms for adverse consequences of treatments/interventions (*adverse events*), and the means of informing NIH of suspension of the research as a result of IRB continuing review.

Database

A *database* is a collection of data that are organized to facilitate search and retrieval of information. Computerized databases are popular because of their storage capacities and the rapidity of search and retrieval. However, not all databases are computerized or need to be. The user determines the logic of the organizational scheme that will best serve *data management needs.

Data Management

Data management refers to operations in place for effectively and systematically collecting, storing, retrieving, and manipulating data. The concept is relevant for all researchers, since the need for a planned data

37

management approach applies to any type of investigation. Qualitative researchers, who tend to amass large quantities of data, stress the importance of designing an effective data management system prior to actual data collection. This organization generally is some combination of paper and computerized filing systems tailored to the needs of the particular research. Other aspects of data management involve procedures that accompany data analysis where data may be broken down (sorted and indexed) via *coding schemes and displayed in visually distinctive ways (e.g., lists, matrices, charts, maps, or diagrams that usually evolve over the course of the study). The aim is to make complex data easier to work with and understand. However, the method should not be allowed to become the master. That is, it is important to make careful, well-reasoned data management choices that <u>facilitate</u> rather than direct the analysis of the data.

See **Computer-Assisted Research.**

Deconstruction

The term *deconstruction* refers to a school of textual analysis and philosophical critique introduced by Jacques Derrida (and identified with a certain circle of literary critics in the 1970s known as the 'Yale School'). Deconstruction is a poststructuralist way of thinking that focuses on complexity, in a critical response to structuralism's focus on discovering universal systems of thought. In other words, deconstructionist thinking assumes that there always is something more that could be communicated by a text (understood broadly as any form of communication, although the written word is the most common type of 'text' subjected to this intense form of interrogation). The objective, then, is to show how the text itself can be made to reveal what it does not, and perhaps cannot or does not need to, say or communicate. To this end, a deconstructive 'reading' or interpretation of a literary text or a theoretical/philosophical position involves an effort to demonstrate how an idea or concept (the dominant discourse or main argument of the text) also contains different, 'decentered,' and contrasting meanings that may be in opposition to one another (e.g., hidden, previously excluded, or silenced *'voices'). Deconstructing various forms of communication to show how they are internally contradictory and incomplete is an intellectual process that involves an appreciation for the subjective and nonuniversal, contextually contingent nature of human experience. Thus, as Tarnas (1991) puts it, Derrida's deconstructionism challenges "the attempt to establish a secure meaning in any text" (p. 398). The multiple possibilities that exist for directing discussion on a given topic provide the means by which a deconstruction of a particular work may demonstrate how no single text or interpretation can ever completely and conclusively address an experience in its totality. However, deconstruction, or taking apart and reconstructing the messages within a text, does not mean that the text is necessarily faulty for failing to deal with every contingency. Rather, the thought behind the process is that knowledge about something involves knowing that there always is something more than can or may need to be known; and what a text does not say as well as what it does say are of equal importance.

See **Poststructuralism** and **Structuralism.**

Deductive Reasoning

Deductive reasoning is a way of thinking (a logical mental process) that begins with premises about a phenomenon and systematically formulates a conclusion that must necessarily follow. That is, the conclusion is dependent upon the premises:

(premise)	all A is B
(premise)	all C is A
(conclusion)	all C is B

The format is fixed, and therefore if the premises are faulty, the conclusion will be faulty as well. A deductive research strategy begins with a general theory or set of abstract propositions that explains how concepts of interest are related. To see if the explanations offered can be verified through empirical observation, a hypothesis is developed and concepts are operationalized by indicating the observations that will generate appropriate empirical data for testing the hypothesis (also called the hypothetico-deductive method). Deductive reasoning is closely associated with physical science (e.g., physics and chemistry) and with mathematics. Some researchers believe that social/human sciences likewise should favor deductive approaches. But there are few instances of strictly deductive approaches to inquiry. It is important to understand that theorists and researchers in these disciplines use both deduction and induction in their work.

See **Inductive Reasoning** and **Theory.**

Degrees of Freedom

Degrees of freedom is a technical term associated with sampling distributions such as t, F, and chi-square that are used in various tests of statistical significance. The number of degrees of freedom is one of the two reference points in tables for those distributions (level of significance is the other) that are found in the backs of just about all statistics books and some nursing research texts.

There are several ways of thinking about degrees of freedom, ranging from 'something you need to carry out certain statistical tests' to 'the number of unconstrained observations.' Formulas for the number of degrees of freedom for a particular test vary considerably from one context to another, but they typically involve the sample size(s) and/or the number of variables.

This is a very difficult term to understand, but not to use. See Munro (2001) or any other good statistics book for further explanation.

See **Test of Significance.**

De-Identified/Limited Data Set

A *de-identified data set* is one that does not contain any of the 18 'identifiers' (names, codes, or any information that could link individuals with the data) defined by U.S. federal law as *protected health information,* which means that its use and disclosure is not subject to *HIPAA* regulations. (It does not mean that data collection procedures are not subject to *Institutional Review Board [IRB] regulations, which apply to all research.) In instances where some protected data are important to a study, a *limited data set* allows for the sharing of certain information fields, such as birth dates, admission/discharge dates, and zip codes that may be critical to the data analysis, but excludes all direct identifiers of the individual or others, such as family members or care providers, as defined by HIPAA. In these circumstances, in order to obtain or share the data, the researcher must enter into a *data use agreement* with health care entities whose standard transactions are covered by HIPAA. This is a formal document that stipulates the conditions governing the disclosure of *protected health information (PHI)* by a 'covered entity' (health care plan, provider, or clearinghouse) and restrictions on its use by a researcher as a limited data set for research purposes (e.g., that the data cannot be disclosed, reused, or used in a way other than that described in the agreement). The *minimum necessary standard* governs covered entities' disclosures and researchers' uses of limited data sets. Part of HIPAA protection is that only the minimum of what is needed to accomplish the research activity may be released. Therefore, research protocols submitted for IRB approval and requests for limited data sets under data use agreements must carefully specify all the data that will need to be collected.

See **HIPAA** and **Protected Health Information (PHI).**

Deletion

Deletion is one way of coping with missing-data problems (the other is imputation). There are two kinds of deletion strategies—listwise and pairwise. In listwise deletion all of the data for a 'case' (a person, hospital, or whatever) are deleted from further analysis if any of the data for that 'case' are absent. In pairwise deletion only the data for the variable(s) that have any 'missingness' are deleted.

For example, if a survey instrument consisting of 100 items is employed in a particular study and a respondent omits just one of those items, with listwise deletion all of the data for that respondent are omitted. That is, of course, very wasteful of data, but it is a 'conservative' strategy. With pairwise deletion, the only deletion is the observation for that item for that respondent (it is really not a deletion since the data for that item were never provided), leaving all the rest of the data for that respondent available for any analyses that do not involve that particular item.

See **Imputation** and **Missing Data.**

Delphi Technique

The *Delphi technique* is a method for obtaining expert opinion on a topic, for example, priorities in nursing research. It employs multiple 'rounds' or 'waves' of questionnaires, with each round utilizing information gathered during previous rounds, in an attempt to converge toward group consensus. It can best be thought of as intermediate between intensive interviewing and traditional survey research.

See Hardy et al. (2004) for an example of an application of the Delphi technique.

Dependability

See **Trustworthiness Criteria.**

Dependent Samples

Dependent samples are samples that are 'paired,' 'matched,' or 'correlated' in some manner. The pairing can arise by virtue of the fact that the samples consist of the same people (or hospitals, thermometers, or whatever) measured on the dependent variable on more than one occasion. Alternatively, the samples may consist of different subjects who have been matched pairwise on the basis of one or more variables known or thought to be related to the dependent variable and are measured simultaneously on the dependent variable. The former situation occurs most often in nonexperimental longitudinal research and in 'repeated-measures' experimental designs. The latter situation is common in 'randomized-block' experimental designs, where each 'block' is a pair of twins, a set of persons with identical or near-identical IQ scores, or the like.

Example: In studying the relative effectiveness of two types of aspirin regarding headache relief, a sample of n adults might be rank-ordered according to age, with one of the two oldest persons randomly assigned to Drug A and the other assigned to Drug B, one member of the next oldest pair randomly assigned to Drug A and the other to Drug B, and so on down through the youngest pair. The two samples would be dependent because they are matched on age.

D

Dependent Variable

The *dependent variable* in a research study is the variable that is of principal interest to the investigator, that is, the variable that really 'counts.' It is in contrast to the independent variable(s) that is (are) known or thought to be at least predictive if not actually causative of the dependent variable.

There is nothing special about *one* independent variable and *one* dependent variable. It is not unusual for a study, especially a nonexperimental study, to have as many as 10 or even 20 independent variables. An occasional study may also employ multiple dependent variables.

A given variable is not automatically relegated to one role or the other. The same measure that is used as the dependent variable in a particular study might very well serve as an independent variable in another study. Polit and Beck (2004) illustrate that point in the following way:

> a study might examine the effects of nurses' contraceptive counseling (the independent variable) on unwanted births (the dependent variable). Another study might investigate the effect of unwanted births (the independent variable) on the incidence of child abuse (the dependent variable) (p. 31).

Example: In a study of the effect of stress on depression, the dependent variable is depression, which may be influenced by stress. Depression is the problem; stress may be symptomatic of, and/or lead to, depression.

Descriptive Research

Descriptive research is a type of quantitative research that is usually preliminary to more controlled experimental or correlational research. It provides a knowledge base when little is known about a phenomenon or when such things as clarification of a situation, classification of information, or description of subject characteristics will aid refinement of the research problem, formulation of hypotheses, or design of data collection and analysis procedures. Surveys and many kinds of interview and observational studies (comparative, cross-sectional, longitudinal) are examples of descriptive research.

Descriptive research is not in the same domain as qualitative research. Qualitative research traditions (which are discussed individually in this dictionary) use descriptive techniques in service to the development of complex interpretive explanations. However, there <u>are</u> qualitative descriptive research studies of lesser complexity for which description rather than interpretation is the end product. They may have overtones of and use similar methods as traditional types of qualitative studies but they "involve a kind of interpretation that is low-inference" and less abstract than studies with an "interpretive spin" (Sandelowski, 2000, pp. 335–336).

There are many examples of classical types of descriptive studies in the nursing literature. See, for example, Börjesson, Paperin, and Lindell (2004), Hendel, Fradkin, and Kidron (2004), Herrington, Olomu, and Geller (2004), Hudson, Kirksey, and Holzemer (2004), Kaasalainen and Crook (2004), and Rowe and Fehrenbach (2004). Some studies use qualitative methods/approaches. See, for example, Jansen and von Sadovszky (2004), Plach, Stevens, and Moss (2004), and Uys (2003).

Descriptive Statistics

Descriptive statistics is the branch of statistics that is concerned with the summarization of data. The data may be for an entire population or for a sample.

Included under descriptive statistics are frequency distributions (the usual starting point for summarizing data), measures of central tendency (means, medians, modes), measures of variability (ranges, variances, standard deviations), measures of relationship (especially correlation coefficients), and various graphical techniques for displaying data.

For sample data, descriptive statistics are often used to highlight certain features of the data that will be the basis for making inferences from sample to population. However, when the data are for an entire population, the sole concern is with descriptive statistics, as there is no statistical inference to be made that goes beyond the data in hand.

Example: A sample survey of attitudes of student nurses toward homosexuality would have a very heavy descriptive statistical component, with frequency distributions for each item and each pair of items. Inferences regarding various population parameters might also be made, but the interpretation of the results of the survey will depend largely on the description of the sample data.

Design

In the broadest sense of the term, *design* refers to the overall approach that is used to answer specific questions and achieve the stated purpose of a research project. Clinical trials, correlational research, ethnographic field studies, grounded theory, and phenomenological investigations are just a small number of examples of generic types of research designs. The purpose of the research and the specific research question guide the choice of a research design. For example, a researcher wishing to test a cause-and-effect relationship between anxiety and academic achievement of student nurses should choose an experimental design in which, ideally, some student nurses are randomly assigned to an anxiety-provoking condition and others are not. If experimentation is impossible or impractical, a measure of anxiety and a measure of achievement could be correlated with one another. A researcher also could choose an ethnographic design to examine the cultural context of nursing education, a grounded theory approach to understand how students manage the educational experience, or a phenomenological design to gain some perspective of what the experience is like. Questions, then, might be related to the meaning of anxiety (as manifested in student subcultures or experienced at a highly personal individual level) or how student nurses respond to and manage anxiety-provoking situations. Such study designs could lead to theories or hypotheses about the nature of or circumstances surrounding student nurse anxiety and its possible relationship to academic achievement.

In a narrower sense of the term, *design* applies to the portion of a research investigation that is concerned with specific methodological issues such as those of sampling, operationalization of theoretical constructs, data collection and data analysis procedures, and approaches to assure that standards of quality associated with the particular design (e.g., accuracy, reliability, credibility) are met. Often, in qualitative studies, the design evolves as the research progresses. For example, the analysis that occurs concurrently with data collection may lead to new questions and different sampling strategies as insights and/or informational categories are formed and developed. However, in quantitative research, design details are not intended to be adjusted once the research is underway.

Determinism

Determinism is the philosophical theory that all events, including human thoughts and actions, are determined by prior occurrences and the operation of natural laws. Strict determinism disavowed the possibility of random events and free will (human agency). Softer versions allow for uncertainty and see free will and determinism as compatible. In social/human science research the term is problematic when used as a pejorative. However, ongoing scientific interests in causality, based on assumptions that some things can be predicted (and, perhaps, controlled), are, by their nature, deterministic.

See **Explanation** and **Causality.**

Dialectic

Dialectic is from the Greek word that means *to converse*. It refers to a style of reasoning, the act of interpretation, or a conversational form of argument/explanation. The dynamic of the dialectic in hermeneutic interpretation is one of question and answer. In critical theory, the dialectic occurs in logically reasoned sequences of contradiction and synthesis with reconciliation of contradictions producing new contradictions. Thus, in the critical theory sense, *dialectics* (or *dialectical analysis*) is a method for systematically weighing and seeking to resolve real or apparent contradictory ideas. See Romyn's (2000) discussion of dialectical analysis as it relates to emancipatory pedagogy in nursing education.

See **Critical Theory** and **Hermeneutics.**

Dialogue

Dialogue, in qualitative inquiry, is a metaphor for the ways in which researchers engage in overlapping (simultaneously occurring) conversations (both internal reflective dialogue and dialogue with others). Embedded in the metaphor are a number of philosophical ideas about knowing and being, the nature of dialogue, and the structures that mediate communication. For example, *dialogue* in Gadamer's (1900–2002) philosophy of *dialogical hermeneutics* is not a method, but a way to think about how one may be able to come to an understanding of anything with which one is concerned. Thus, what is characteristic of a dialogue oriented toward understanding is a positive, creative 'fusion of horizons' where one comes to an understanding (i.e., "whereby [one's] horizon is enlarged and enriched") by being open to the other's point of view (Bernstein, 1983, p. 143). Martin Buber's (1878–1965) *dialogical hermeneutics* also is a philosophy that accounts for the relationships that pertain between Self and Other (i.e., I—It and I—Thou relationships), where choice between the two types of relationships is determined by the way in which Self interprets Other. However, Habermas (1929–   ) "emphasizes . . . societal barriers that systematically distort . . . dialogue" (Bernstein, p. 190). For critical theorists, dialogue is inevitably subject to power and distortion while, at the same time, there is the belief that through dialogue persons have an opportunity to develop a critical understanding of oppression and the means to overcome it. Thus, dialogue is central to the practice of researchers working in interpretive and critical traditions, but what they make of it (philosophical stance) and how they use (engage with) it may vary.

See **Critical Theory** and **Hermeneutics.**

Dichotomy

A *dichotomy* is a nominal variable that consists of just two categories.

Dichotomies are very common in nursing research, particularly as far as independent variables are concerned, because research questions regarding the relationships between sex (a male/female dichotomy) and depression, smoking behavior (a smoke/don't smoke dichotomy) and lung cancer, and the like, are of considerable interest. They are so popular that researchers often make the mistake of throwing away valuable data to get a dichotomy, for example, by collapsing age into two categories (say, under 65 years and over 65 years) rather than keeping it as a continuum when studying its relationship with some dependent variable such as pulse rate.

Although dichotomies are nominal variables, they can be treated like interval variables in statistical calculations because the difference between the values assigned to the two categories constitutes a 'unit' of measurement, however arbitrary, that is constant throughout the scale (it *is* the scale).

Example: Type of treatment (experimental/control) is the classic case of a dichotomy. In an experiment we are always interested in the relationship between that variable and the dependent variable serving as a measure of the outcome of the experiment.

Dimensional Analysis

Schatzman (1991) had earlier developed *dimensional analysis* as a specific technique to help novice researchers learn how to do analysis in grounded theory research. (This was an expansion on the ways in which Glaser and Strauss had described 'analysis.') "Strauss and Corbin (1990) build on his notion" by encouraging researchers to develop categories in terms of their properties (characteristics) and dimensions (location of properties along a continuum) during initial open *coding (Charmaz, 2000, p. 516). For a dimensional analysis research exemplar of an exploration of nurses' clinical reasoning, see Kools, McCarthy, Durham, and Robrecht (1996).

Caron and Bowers (2000) also have introduced dimensional analysis as a method for conducting a *concept analysis, illustrating its use with an example of an analysis of nurse/client relationships. They discuss how dimensional analysis may be used "to uncover unquestioned assumptions about a given concept . . . and to identify important questions and inconsistencies that need to be addressed" (p. 316). For another example of this in the nursing literature, see Shearer's (2002) dimensional analysis to clarify the concept of protection "which has a commonly understood definition but is used inconsistently in research literature. The article critiques a situation-specific theory of protection [and] compares conceptual literature to identify inconsistencies in use" (p. 65).

See **Grounded Theory.**

Discourse Analysis

Discourse analysis is a general term for a variety of approaches, some of which involve (a) the interpretive analysis of recorded talk (Silverman, 2000) and others that involve (b) the critical analysis of *ideologies that underlie language use and social discourse. The interpretive analysis of interviews, texts, and transcripts focuses on the characteristics of social discourse in everyday interaction, in terms of interactive meanings and/or the conversational structure of talk (Gubrium & Holstein, 2000). It is associated with methods of sociolinguistics, ethnomethodology, and communication studies. Critical discourse analysis focuses on the assumptions that structure ways of talking and thinking about a given topic and the social functions that the discourse serves. For example, Michel Foucault (1926–1984), whose work is closely associated with this approach, used the term *power/knowledge* to express how "power operates in and through discourse as the other face of knowledge" (Gubrium & Holstein, p. 494). That is, knowledge is not 'truth' apart from power (represented by some dominant ideology) with which it is entangled. Consequently, 'truth' must be seen as 'socially constructed' in ways that further and support the aims and needs of the dominant ideology. Discourse analysis also is linked with *poststructuralist approaches and *deconstruction. For examples in the nursing literature, see Baggens (2004), Fealy (2004), Georges (2003), Georges and McGuire (2004), P. K. Hardin (2003), Kramer (2002), and P. Powers (2003).

See **Ethnomethodology** and **Critical Theory.**

D

Discriminant Analysis

Discriminant analysis is a type of multivariate analysis in which two or more criterion groups defined according to some dependent variable are contrasted regarding two or more independent variables, to determine the extent to which those independent variables are capable of 'discriminating' among the groups as far as prediction of group membership is concerned.

Discriminant analysis was used by Rizzuto, Bostrom, Suter, and Chenitz (1994) in their study of nurses' involvement in research activities.

See **Multivariate Analysis.**

Discriminant Validity

Discriminant validity is a type of construct validity. If there is *not* a strong relationship between a particular measure and one or more other measures that are alleged to operationalize different but easily confusable constructs, then the given measure is said to possess discriminant validity.

See **Validity.**

Double-Blind Study

A *double-blind study* is an experiment in which neither the experimenter nor the subject knows who is getting which treatment. (*Somebody,* usually the researcher who designs and analyzes the experiment, has to know or the data could never get sorted out.)

The purpose of the double-blind approach is to avoid the confounding of the actual treatment effect with any extraneous factors that may be associated with the mere knowledge of treatment identification, such as lack of motivation on the part of subjects who know that they have been given a placebo or the giving of additional encouragement to experimental subjects by the experimenter.

There are also 'single-blind' experiments in which the subjects do not know which treatment they are receiving but the experimenters do.

Example: An experimental study of the effectiveness of any sort of pill, such as the every-other-day aspirin in the Physicians' Health Study, often employs the double-blind technique. In that study the physicians were both subjects and experimenters, as they self-administered the pills that were mailed to them and they did not know whether they were getting the aspirin or the placebo.

Dummy Variable

A *dummy variable* is a special kind of dichotomy that uses the numbers 0 and 1 as codes to represent the two categories of the variable.

Dummy variables are most commonly used in conjunction with regression analysis, for natural dichotomies such as sex and type of treatment, and for artificial dichotomies arising from the coding of multicategoried nominal variables such as political affiliation and eye color. Dummy coding is one of the three popular ways of coding; the other two are contrast coding and effect coding. It is called dummy coding because the numbers used for coding purposes (0 and 1) have nothing to do with none or one of anything, and are, therefore, "dummy" numbers.

Example: When investigating the relationship between attitude toward abortion (a continuous score of some kind) and religious affiliation (say a four-categoried nominal variable: Catholic, Protestant, Jew, Other), the religious affiliation variable might be transformed into three dummy variables X_1 (1 = Catholic, 0 = non-Catholic), X_2 (1 = Protestant, 0 = non-Protestant), and X_3 (1 = Jew, 0 = non-Jew), and a multiple regression analysis with those three independent variables and one dependent variable (the attitude score) would be carried out. A fourth dummy variable is both unnecessary and redundant, because the "Others" are uniquely identified by a coding of 0 on X_1, X_2, and X_3.

E

Effect Size

Effect size, is a measure of an effect postulated in the alternative hypothesis, as contrasted with the 'no effect' null hypothesis. It is usually defined as the difference between two population means divided by their common standard deviation. The term is a crucial concept in the determination of sample size for quantitative research.

In the meta-analysis literature, effect size has a different meaning. There is the *actual* effect obtained in a particular study, rather than a hypothesized effect.

The 'effect' is not necessarily causal, no matter what the context.

Example: A researcher might hypothesize that the RN/LPN difference in salary (the effect size for professional preparation) is .5 standard deviations, that is, half of the standard deviation for the salary variable.

Emic/Etic

The term *emic* relates to the perspectives that are shared and understood by members of a particular culture, the 'insiders,' in contrast to the perspectives of the culture that nonmember observers, the 'outsiders,' may have, which are called *etic* perspectives. The contrast between 'insider' and 'outsider' (emic vs. etic) perspectives is important in ethnographic research.

See Ethnography.

Empirical Indicator/Referent

An *empirical indicator* or *referent* is an observable object, property, or event that is linked to a concept or construct in a theory as a way of defining it, or can be operationalized as a research variable for theory testing.

See Theory and Operational Definition.

Empirical Knowing

Empirical knowing in nursing is concerned with scientific inquiry, that is, theory building and research (Carper, 1978). Chinn and Kramer (2004) describe activities involved in the creation of empiric knowledge (i.e., knowledge based on sensory experience) as theory development (explaining and structuring empiric phenomena), theory evaluation (describing and reflecting on empiric theory), and empirical research (investigating, replicating and validating empiric knowledge).

See **Empirical Research** and **Patterns of Knowing.**

Empirical Research

The term *empirical research* applies to <u>any</u> scientific study (qualitative or quantitative using either inductive or hypothetico-deductive processes of reasoning) in which some sort of evidence is obtained through methods that rely on the senses (i.e., direct or indirect observation). The evidence is in turn called **data*. Empirical research is often confused with experimental research; the latter is a subset of the former. Empirical research also should not be confused with strict empiricism, a theoretical perspective/paradigm that posited that the <u>only</u> legitimate approach to knowledge was through verifiable empirical observations (not reason or interpretation).

See **Experiment, Research,** and **Empiricism.**

Empiricism

Empiricism belongs to a family of theoretical perspectives whose view is that scientific knowledge is advanced by systematic study of objective reality that may be experienced through the senses. *Strict empiricism* posited that sense experience is the <u>sole source</u> of scientific knowledge, resulting in hard facts that are verifiable through methods of observation and experimentation and are free from spontaneous ideas, a priori thought, and subjective interpretation. Drawing on the strict empiricism of Aristotle (384–322 BC), this approach to scientific investigation was popularized by Francis Bacon (1561–1626) and was promoted by what became known as the British empiricist school of philosophy. Leading figures were John Locke (1632–1704), George Berkeley (1685–1753), and David Hume (1711–1776). The rise of empiricism was associated with the rising importance of experimental science as something distinct from pure mathematics. Over time, there have been various versions of empiricist/positivist thinking (see below).

See **Positivism, Logical Positivism, Logical Empiricism, Postempiricism,** and **Postpositivism**

Endogenous Variable

In path analysis an *endogenous variable* is any variable whose causal determination is of interest to the researcher and the nature of that causation is hypothesized in the path model.

See **Path Analysis.**

Epidemiological Research

Epidemiological research is the science of determining the extent and causes of disease in human populations (i.e., *risk factors) and their natural history and progression, as well as evaluating approaches to prevent and control disease (e.g., the efficacy, effectiveness, and/or cost-benefit of health care screening and treatment programs). Epidemiological findings are often used to inform health care policy and decision making. Causal inferences in epidemiological research are almost never based on controlled experiments, as the kinds of independent variables of principal concern in such research usually are not manipulable. The 'case-control' type of retrospective research is an approach often employed, as is prospective research using a cohort design. An example of epidemiological research on a nursing problem is illustrated by Zimmer, N. Watson, and Treat's (1984) first population-based documentation of behavioral problems among residents of nursing homes.

Epistemology

The term *epistemology* refers to the study or a philosophy of knowledge that involves an understanding of its nature, origin, and scope as well as justification of knowledge claims (i.e., its reliability and limits). It is the philosophical underpinning of different theoretical perspectives and methodologies that guide scientific research.

See **Objectivism**, **Subjectivism**, and **Constructivism/Constructionism.**

EQS

See **Structural Equation Modeling.**

Error

The term *error* is used in several contexts in nursing research but usually does not refer to making a mistake.

One of the most common contexts is in the analysis of variance, where error refers to within-treatment variance attributable to individual differences among subjects who receive the same experimental treatment, but who do not get the same score on the dependent variable. Another context is in sampling, where a particular statistic for a sample is not exactly equal to the corresponding population parameter because of chance factors associated with the drawing of the sample. A third context is classical measurement theory, where a measurement error is defined as the difference between an 'obtained' score and a 'true' score.

The one context in which the term 'error' actually means 'mistake' is in statistical hypothesis-testing. A 'Type I error' is the rejection of a true null hypothesis; a 'Type II error' is the failure to reject a false null hypothesis.

E

Essences

Essences are the internal meaning structures of a phenomenon that are grasped intuitively through the study of the ways in which they manifest themselves in lived experience (van Manen, 1990, p. 10).

See **Phenomenology.**

Ethical Knowing

Ethical knowing is knowledge of the moral basis of practice expressed by values, principles, obligations, rules, and codes (Carper, 1978). Analysis and generation of ethical knowledge is accomplished through processes of dialogue and argument. Dialogue occurs over time as arguments for various perspectives on ethical issues are shared through the literature. "It ultimately is through these processes . . . that ethical knowledge forms will achieve a legitimacy in relation to practice" (Chinn & Kramer, 2004, p. 174).

See **Patterns of Knowing.**

Ethnography

Ethnography is both a process and a product. As a process it involves an attitude inclined toward learning from rather than studying persons in order to understand their lifeways and *worldview in cultural context. Ethnographers analyze *emic (participants' 'insider') and etic (the researcher's 'outsider') perspectives together in order to compare understandings and to capture differences between what people say and what they do.

An implicit principle in ethnographic research is that the researcher can only capture an 'insider' point of view through some degree of immersion in the *culture.

Cultural understanding is gained through *fieldwork, a method that requires the researcher's presence in study participants' environments—participating in everyday life, systematically recording and validating observations, and conducting formal and informal interviews. *Participant observation is the central technique in ethnographic fieldwork. It involves researcher engagement in ordinary everyday activities for the explicit purpose of systematically observing/experiencing their nature, the people who participate, and the context in which they take place. In-depth interviewing is an adjunct to participant observation that employs a conversational style to draw individuals out and allow them to talk at great length about a topic; but it is multifaceted. It involves different combinations of open-ended, semi-structured, and structured interview formats to ensure cross-validation and informational consistency across participants as well as to pursue new ideas as directed by the data analysis, which occurs simultaneously with data collection.

As a product, an 'ethnography' may be one of many types (e.g., classical/comprehensive descriptions of a culture, biographical, autobiographical, narrative, interpretive, critical). Researchers also can represent "the same material in many different ways, using different formats, styles, and genres" (Tedlock, 2000, p. 459). See B. A. Powers (2001, 2003a, 2003b, 2005b) for examples of and discussion about the use of different representational styles for the same data set; see Crabtree (2003), Dombeck (2003), Kayser-Jones (2002), Mohr (2004), Tzeng and Lipson (2004), and Ward-Griffin, Bol, Hay, & Dashnay (2003) for additional examples of ethnographic nursing research.

Ethnomethodology

Ethnomethodology (literally, 'people's methods') is a branch of sociology created by Harold Garfinkel in the 1940s. Its aim is to study how people 'do' everyday things (initiate telephone conversations, walk, invite laughter, and deal with unexpected disruptions) for the purpose of "document[ing] how they concretely construct and sustain social entities, such as gender, self, and family" (Gubrium & Holstein, 2000, p. 490).

Ethnomethodologists gather empirical data through observation, conversation, and video or audio recording, not to describe everyday life but to theorize about the ways in which people use taken-for-granted rules in social situations to manage and structure their lives. Ethnomethodology reached the height of its productivity in the late 1960s and early '70s. However, internal debates in sociology hindered its spread; and, although some nurses have a background in this methodology, it has not been influential in nursing research.

Ethnoscience

Ethnoscience (semantic *ethnography) is a method of analyzing culture to ascertain the system of knowledge and beliefs as it is reflected in native language categories. It focuses on emic ('insider') data. Results are often in the form of taxonomies or semantic network diagrams.

See **Emic/Etic.**

Evaluation Research

Evaluation research is a term that is applied to a wide spectrum of investigative activities that employ research methods and a problem-solving process to meet program or practice needs. *Quality assurance (QA)* and *continuous quality improvement (CQI)* are other terms used for these activities carried out in institutional settings. (It is important for institutions to distinguish between internal QA and human subjects research activities to determine when *Institutional Review Board review is necessary.)

The term *evaluation* applies broadly to processes for assessing and judging the quality of care or services rendered. In the health sciences this is a very important—and legally mandated—activity that may focus on structure (e.g., the nature of resources and personnel), process (e.g., the nature of staff activities), or outcome (e.g., the result[s]/effect[s] of a particular type of care or service on recipients). The usual approach involves identifying criteria or behavioral objectives that represent the goals, valued practice models, or desired outcomes; setting a "standard" that represents the level (often expressed as a percentage) at which each criterion must be met in order to judge the program, policy, procedure, practice, and so forth as 'effective' or of 'acceptable quality'; employing data and analysis methods designed to answer the question about the extent of compliance with the standard set for each criterion (this could involve experimental or nonexperimental methodologies); implementing corrective changes if indicated; and setting the cycle in motion again by evaluating the results. (A standard must not be confused with a norm. A norm is 'what is'; a standard is 'what should be.') Evaluation can be formative or summative. Formative evaluation allows for continuous feedback and adjustment of interventions or programs as they progress. The emphasis is on monitoring them as they develop. Summative evaluation focuses on how a program or practice influences the outcomes that the study seeks to measure, that is, how effective it is in meeting stated objectives or standards. Note: The above description illustrates the considerable overlap between the broad definition of *evaluation research* and *health services research* (see entry for *health services research*).

The following examples of evaluation research from the nursing literature also mention **stakeholders,* an important consideration in evaluation research that seeks to involve the perspectives of persons most invested in and/or affected by the programs or practices that are the focus of the evaluation. See Ansari, Phillips, and Zwi (2004), Gerrish and Griffith (2004), Hall (2004), and Scholes et al. (2004).

See **Health Services Research.**

Evidence

The meaning of *evidence* as it pertains to knowledge development in nursing (or any discipline) is part of a debate that has been going on since ancient times about what is to count as knowledge. There are many variations on this theme, but in short, there are two major camps. One camp is established in a **positivist tradition of science influenced by cultural strains of **modernism. A recent article in *Worldviews on Evidence-Based Nursing* articulates this view very clearly: "Modern health science rests on an explicitly positivist base . . . [And] the evidence-based practice movement asserts a particular kind of truth claim in its advocacy of evidence as the basis for practice—the appeal to science" (Scott-Findlay & Pollock, 2004, pp. 93–94). Thus, in the evidence-based practice movement (which is how the term *evidence* is invoked in this long-standing conversation), proponents of this view differentiate between *evidence* as tangible *empirical research findings, subjected to rigorous testing to reduce *bias and increase *generalizability, versus *knowledge* as personally constructed interpretations/understandings that are necessarily biased and nongeneralizable. Scott-Findlay and Pollock nicely articulate an extreme, yet arguably dominant *worldview of evidence-based practice:

> We urge the restriction of the term *evidence* to research findings, and while acknowledging the importance of other influences on the clinical decision-making process, it is argued that they are not evidence . . . The time has come to value personal experience and clinical expertise for what they are—they should not have to be 'disguised' as types of evidence for them to be deemed of any value (p. 96).

The other camp is established in *interpretivist and *constructionist traditions of science (a term appropriated by 'positivist science' and reclaimed by 'human scientists') influenced by the cultural strains of *poststructuralism and *postmodernism (although this oversimplifies the eclecticism and diversity of worldviews that characterize this other side of the conversation). Thus, some nurse theorists argue against a solely empirical model of *evidence* and advocate for evidence-based nursing practice that draws more broadly upon a postmodern worldview (J. Watson, 1995, 1999) to develop a *holistic interpretation of the different kinds of *evidence* required for nursing practice, based on an integration of Carper's (1978) four diverse *patterns of knowing (Chinn & Kramer, 2004; Fawcett et al., 2001). The following qualitative researcher viewpoint (Powers of Powers and Knapp) is an extension of these ideas and an expansion of Scott-Findlay and Pollock's (2004) understanding of what may constitute 'research findings.'

Evidence, in lay language, most often refers to the grounds, justification, or reasons for a decision or conclusion. What <u>counts</u> as evidence depends on the question that is asked; and what evidence <u>matters</u> depends on the questions one cares about. What counts and what matters represent related but different concerns about <u>questions</u>.

In *evidence-based practice (EBP), the questions most commonly asked are those originally defined by evidence-based medicine (EBM). They are (a) *diagnosis questions* about the degree to which a particular test is reliable and clinically useful; (b) *prognosis questions* about a patient's future life span and quality of life if (s)he chooses a particular treatment option; (c) *therapy questions* about what treatment, if any, to give a patient and outcomes of treatment options; and (d) *harm questions* about the relationship between a disease or other condition and a

E

possible cause. Of these, therapy/treatment questions are the most likely to be addressed by evidence-based nursing intervention studies; and what counts as evidence is determined by the correspondence of the research question to some level on an evidence hierarchy, the gold standard of which is the randomized controlled clinical trial. However, there are other questions that matter to nurses; and what counts as evidence in relation to them does not logistically correspond to this evidence hierarchy.

Other questions that matter to nurses are (a) *context questions* about the personal, ethical, social, and cultural circumstances within which clinical care decisions are made and implemented; (b) *response questions* about how persons process and manage health issues in their everyday lives, including encounters with systems and providers; and (c) *meaning questions* about how persons deal with health/illness concerns in terms of what they know, how they feel, and what they believe. What counts as evidence is determined by the correspondence of the research question to qualitative research traditions with diverse theoretical perspectives and methodologies that are nonhierarchical. In EBP terms, context, response, and meaning questions could be background or foreground questions, depending on the circumstances; but that may not be the best way to think about them. Qualitative researchers might be more likely to favor holistic interpretations of how various types of evidence-based knowledge 'fit' a situation, consistent with the ideas of the above-cited nurse theorists (i.e., J. Watson, Fawcett et al., Chinn & Kramer).

Rycroft-Malone and Stetler (2004) offer a moderating response (most specifically in the form of a commentary on Scott-Findlay and Pollock's, 2004, article) to what will likely be an ongoing conversation in nursing between the two camps. They note that "evidence can be derived from multiple sources of knowledge," make reference to "many hierarchies of evidence" and suggest that Scott-Findlay and Pollock appear to be "coming from an epidemiological perspective" (historical foundation of evidence-based practice) where "a common assumption is that evidence is research evidence and more specifically from the quantitative tradition" (Rycroft-Malone & Stetler, p. 99). In summation, they characterize arguments over what constitutes legitimate forms of evidence in health care as the "challenge" before us regarding how the multiple influences that impact on clinical decision making are to be "weighted" and, in addition, "how these influences are blended and to what extent they positively impact patient outcomes" (p. 100).

See **Evidence-Based Practice.**

Evidence-Based Practice (EBP)

Evidence-based practice (EBP) is the general term for an approach to clinical problem solving that has a number of variants (e.g., evidence-based nursing [EBN] and evidence-based health care [EBHC]). It began as an undergraduate teaching model (evidence-based medicine/EBM) pioneered by David Sackett, Gordon Guyatt, and others at McMaster University, Hamilton, Ontario, Canada. Guided by processes of clinical epidemiology, it gained visibility via a landmark article in *JAMA* (Evidence-Based Medicine Working Group, 1992) and a weeklong workshop on teaching EBM at a newly established Centre for Evidence-Based Medicine in Oxford, England, in 1995. The emphasis in EBP is on finding and basing clinical decisions on best research evidence coordinated with clinical expertise and patient values and preferences. (Although it has been compared, at times, to *research utilization,* as discussed in that entry, the two are not the same.)

Process: The EBP process involves four steps. (a) Converting clinical problems into answerable questions involves formulating either general (background) or specific (foreground) questions, such as the following: *Background question*—'What is the effect of tobacco smoking on the circulatory system?' *Foreground question*—'Does clinician counseling result in a higher rate of smoking cessation among smokers in primary care practice than do written materials?' (b) Locating *best evidence with maximum efficiency involves information management skills including, especially, the use of electronic databases. (c) Critically appraising evidence for its validity, importance, and usefulness involves application of specific criteria to determine the methodological rigor, significance, and generalizability of research findings. (d) Integrating this appraisal with clinical expertise and patient values involves considering how research-based best evidence corresponds to clinicians' prior experiences and unique knowledge of both the patient and the situation.

Evolution: The institutional culture of EBP is slowly evolving beyond its historical roots in clinical epidemiology and medicine. It continues to be dominated by an empirical model of evidence that favors questions that lend themselves to quantifiable research approaches. Major emphasis has been placed on holding worldwide workshops, developing centers to promote EBP, and creating materials to help individuals locate best evidence and critically appraise research studies. Material efforts have been in the form of 'user guides' (published as a series in *JAMA*); texts, such as Sackett, Straus, Richardson, Rosenberg, and Haynes (2000) 'bible' on how to practice and teach EBM, Guyatt and Rennie's (2002) updated compilation of the *JAMA* user guide series, and Melnyk and Fineout-Overholt's (2005) *Evidence-Based Practice in Nursing and Healthcare;* journals (e.g., in nursing, *Evidence-Based Nursing* and *Worldviews on Evidence-Based Nursing*); and multiple electronic databases. In addition to traditional bibliographic databases (e.g., MEDLINE and CINAHL) and Internet search systems, sources such as the Cochrane Library, TRIP medical resources database, and the American Colleges of Physicians (ACP) Journal Club (formerly Best Evidence) contain some explicit

E

evidence processing. The Cochrane Library is the source of the world's largest collection of *clinical trials and *meta-analyses of clinical trials. In 1998, the Cochrane Qualitative Methods Network was established for researchers interested in exploring incorporation of qualitative research into Cochrane reviews. However, qualitative studies are less well represented in EBP-focused *systematic reviews; and ways to understand and more routinely include them are underdeveloped. The extent to which they will be included in the future may rest more on 'the questions that matter' to EBP than on the current focus on appraisal guides that serves to skirt the larger issue (see entry on *evidence*). Currently, approaches to *metasynthesis of multiple qualitative research findings appear to be a good way to incorporate knowledge from these approaches into systematic literature reviews that are currently dominated by quantitative research study findings (Powers, B. A., 2005a).

See **Evidence.**

Ex Post Facto Research

Although the term *ex post facto research* is used in a number of different ways in nursing research (some authors equate it with any form of nonexperimental research), it is best thought of as a retrospective type of causal-comparative correlational research.

In ex post facto research one starts with the dependent variable and makes a search into the past for one or more independent variables that may at least partially 'explain' that dependent variable.

Example: The prototypical example of ex post facto research is the investigation of the association between cigarette smoking and lung cancer. Such an investigation most often begins by identifying a group of people who have lung cancer and a comparable group who do not have lung cancer, and proceeds to attempt to determine if the cigarette-smoking history of the two groups differs. If the cancer group has a long history of heavy smoking and the 'control' group (that designation is often used even though the study is *not* an experiment) does not, a case can be made that cigarette smoking is one of the possible causes of lung cancer. It is essential to realize, however, that such evidence does not prove that cigarette smoking is an actual cause, much less the only cause.

Exemplar

An *exemplar* is a specific example (numeric/symbolic formula or word picture) that is representative or typical of some more abstract concept or idea. Sidani, Epstein, and Moritz (2003) used an ongoing multisite study on insomnia as an exemplar in their methods-focused discussion of a theory-driven approach to intervention evaluation. See also Titler's (2004) review and use of four investigations of natural experiments in evidence-based practices as exemplars of translation research.

Exogenous Variable

In path analysis an *exogenous variable* is any variable whose causative determination is external to the path model and is of no interest to the researcher, but whose causal effects on one or more other variables (endogenous variables) is of direct concern.

See **Path Analysis.**

Experiment

An *experiment* is a study that involves manipulation of the principal independent variable, that is, the actual administration of treatments or interventions that comprise the categories of the independent variable. An investigation is made of the effect of the independent variable on the dependent variable.

A *true experiment is characterized by a high degree of control over the unwanted influence of extraneous variables and other factors that could bias the results of the study. The researcher typically investigates the difference on the dependent variable between one group of subjects who get the experimental treatment and another group of subjects who do not. (It sometimes happens that the experimental group and the control group consist of the *same* people, i.e., every person gets *both* the experimental treatment *and* the control treatment, in randomized order. Such designs are called repeated-measures designs.)

In some experiments the dependent variable is measured both before and after the intervention. The measurement taken before the intervention is called a pretest and the measurement taken after the intervention is called a posttest. In other experiments the measurement is taken only after the intervention. The former designs are called, naturally enough, 'pretest-posttest designs,' whereas the latter designs are called 'posttest-only designs.'

In an experiment involving two (or more) independent variables, one may be interested not only in the effect of each of them on the dependent variable but also in the combined effect (interaction) of the independent variables. Experimental designs in which both kinds of effects are tested are called factorial designs.

Example: A study in which one group of nursing students is taught how to administer an injection by Teaching Method A (a film, say) and another group of students is taught by Method B ('hands-on' demonstration using a dummy, say), is an experiment because the principal independent variable (type of teaching method) is actually manipulated by the researcher.

Experimental Group

The *experimental group* is the group that receives the 'treatment' of particular interest to the researcher.

See **Experiment.**

Explanation

Scientific research aims to go beyond description to an *explanation* that is an accounting for or discussion of the cause of a phenomenon or event (very often for the purpose of establishing a basis for predicting its occurrence and controlling/manipulating outcomes). This is an important feature of health science research, where prevention and/or treatment of health concerns (such as pain or disease) are major objectives. Research of any kind will produce explanations in the commonsense use of the term as a reasoned discussion or explication of something. However, in the field of scientific inquiry, what constitutes adequate grounds for an explanation and what kinds of explanations may be privileged over others are much-disputed matters. A classic perspective on the logic of explanation (in terms of its adequacy) is Hempel's covering-law model "officially titled the deductive-nomological (or D-N) model because it envisions explanation as a deductive argument where the premises contain at least one nomological or lawlike empirical generalization" (McErlean, 2000, p. 19). Other probabilistic-statistical models offer formulas for bringing together laws, premises, propositions, and other theory elements in ways that support explanations of causality. The adequacy of different explanatory models and the criteria that argue for superiority of one model/theory over another are continually disputed. Many of these disputes take place within the quantitative camp from whence the theories have sprung. However, despite explanatory research's long-standing association with quantitative research designs, more recently it has been argued that, taken on its own terms and judged by its own criteria, qualitative research may be an equally legitimate and in some cases the best scientific approach to causal explanation (Maxwell, 2004; Roth, 2000). Acceptance of this view involves the realization that interpretive qualitative explanations cannot be understood through deterministic, reductionistic linear models. There also is not unanimity within the qualitative camp, as some interpretivists object to the idea of seeming to move in the direction of developing what may be taken as causal, lawlike theoretical explanations of human/social behavior that they believe is not the manner in which humans should be understood. Rabinow and Sullivan (1979) say:

> . . . as soon as we begin to conduct an inquiry we are caught in a circle [the hermeneutic circle] . . . The only ways out of this circle would be to find simple brute data which everyone could agree on, or to invent a neutral language to describe the data, or both (p. 8).

and C. Taylor (1979) says:

> . . . there is no verification process we can fall back on. We can only continue to offer interpretations (p. 75).

See **Causality, Generalizations, Hermeneutic Circle,** and **Interpretation.**

Exploratory Data Analysis

Exploratory data analysis is a type of statistical analysis that utilizes a special collection of largely graphical descriptive statistics for summarizing research findings.

Included under exploratory data analysis are techniques such as stem-and-leaf diagrams and q-q plots that lend themselves very nicely to modern-day computer technology. (For further details see Tukey, 1977, and three articles by Ferketich and Verran—Ferketich & Verran, 1986; Verran & Ferketich, 1987a, 1987b.)

Example: One of Tukey's popular statistics is the '95% trimmed mean,' which is the mean for a particular variable calculated after the highest 2.5% and the lowest 2.5% of the observations have been deleted (trimmed). The rationale for this is to determine an average that is not affected by extreme data ('outliers') that might otherwise have an undue influence. Such a statistic is routinely reported in statistical 'packages' that include exploratory data analyses.

External Validity

External validity is a synonym for generalizability, which is one of the important goals of most scientific research. The term was coined by Campbell and Stanley (1966) in their classic work on experimental designs. A study is said to have a high degree of external validity if the results of the study can be generalized to people, measuring instruments, and settings other than the ones actually employed in the study itself. Campbell and Stanley discuss a number of 'threats' to the external validity of a research design that might restrict its generalizability, for example, 'reactive arrangements' such as the Hawthorne Effect whereby people who know they are participating in a research study may behave differently from the way they would behave in 'real life.'

'External validity' is actually an unfortunate choice of term for this characteristic of a research investigation, because the root word *validity* is a *measurement* term that may have nothing at all to do with generalizability.

Example: A study of the effect of previous information about patients on the attitudes of student nurses toward those patients would have greater external validity if two sets of descriptions (one favorable, one unfavorable) were randomly distributed to the students without telling them that they were part of a study than if they were told. Such a study might raise some ethical questions, however, because the students would be manipulated without either their knowledge or their consent.

Lincoln and Guba (1985) have described *transferability* as the qualitative research equivalent of external validity. Transferability is demonstrated by information that is sufficient for a reader of the research report to determine whether findings are meaningful when the knowledge is applied in similar types of situations.

See **Generalizations** and **Trustworthiness Criteria.**

Extraneous Variable

An *extraneous variable* is a potentially confounding variable that is not of any particular interest to the researcher but should be controlled if the results of the study are to be interpreted properly.

See **Control.**

F

F test

The *F test* is a test of statistical significance that is usually associated with the analysis of variance.

McDonald et al. (2003) used the F test in conjunction with their one-way analysis of variance in studying the effect of diagnosis on nursing care.

See Test of Significance.

Face Validity

Face validity is a type of content validity in which the 'expert' judgment of the validity of an instrument is provided by the people who are to be measured with the instrument.

See Validity

Factor Analysis

Factor analysis is a statistical procedure for determining the underlying dimensionality of a set of variables.

The variables can be as specific as a collection of test items or as general as a group of physiological measurements. In the former case, the focus is typically on the subscale structure (whether or not there *are* subscales, and if so, *how many* subscales are necessary to describe the construct being measured). In the latter case it is often a matter of trying to cut down the number of variables by arriving at the most 'parsimonious' factor solution.

Most factor analyses are 'exploratory' in that no theoretical expectations are formulated beforehand as to the number or nature of underlying factors. The most common such procedure is the so-called Little-Jiffy technique that involves principal components factor extraction with orthogonal rotation to simple structure of all factors for which the eigenvalues are greater than one. Some factor analyses are 'confirmatory' in that certain hypotheses regarding the number of factors and the factor structure are actually tested in the process of carrying out the analysis. The distinction between exploratory and confirmatory factor analysis is summarized in Munro's (2001) text.

Example: An exploratory factor analysis of a 100-item health behavior inventory might yield two subscales that could be identified as "Beliefs" and "Practices," with some items contributing primarily to the Belief dimension and with other items contributing primarily to the Practices dimension.

For a recent example of factor analysis in nursing research, see Tourangeau and McGilton (2004).

Factorial Design

A *factorial design* is a design that involves two or more independent variables whose main effects and interaction effects are of equal interest in the research. The term is usually associated with experimental research in which the independent variables are actually manipulated by the investigator.

See Interaction Effect and Main Effect.

Feasibility Study

A *feasibility study* is a small-scale study that is undertaken to determine if the design, instrumentation, and analysis for the proposed 'main study' are practicable. The results of such a study are of no concern. The focus is on the extent to which the logistical features of the proposed study are capable of being carried out successfully.

A feasibility study is similar to a pilot study, although the latter type of study is often used to gather some preliminary evidence regarding the validity and reliability of the measuring instruments.

Example: A main study in which very expensive and/or invasive instrumentation is to be employed should be preceded by a feasibility study whose principal objective is to see if research subjects will be willing to be 'attached' to various devices, how much time it will take to gather the data, and the like.

See Chang (2004) for a recent example of a feasibility study.

Feminist Research

Feminist research involves an epistemological stance, or theoretical perspective, that gives direction to the many forms of inquiry in this field (both *qualitative and *quantitative in nature). The goal is to entertain a critical dialogue that focuses on women's experiences in historical, cultural, and socioeconomic perspective. Lorber (2001) organizes the multiple theories that guide feminist research into several typologies. These

F

typologies are: (a) gender reform feminisms (liberal, Marxist, and post-colonial) that want to change social structures that disadvantage women; (b) gender resistance feminisms (radical, lesbian, psychoanalytic, and standpoint theories) that examine the sources of sexual oppression and men's violence toward women; and (c) gender rebellion feminisms (multicultural, men's, social construction, postmodern, and queer theories) that attack the gender system, arguing that the categorization of men vs. women needs to be expanded for the betterment of theory, research, and politics. See also Tong's (1998) introduction to the varieties of feminist thinking (e.g., liberal, Marxist, radical, psychoanalytic, existentialist and postmodern feminists).

Olesen (2000) describes "major strands within contemporary feminist research" as

(a) writing by women of color . . . (critical [studies] that problematize not only the construction of women of color in relation to whiteness but unremitting whiteness itself), . . . (b) postcolonial feminist thought (pointing to issues of globalization, such as unsafe and exploitive working conditions . . . and the international sex trade) . . . (c) lesbian research and queer theory . . . (d) disabled women . . . (e) standpoint theory and research [an engaged vision and understanding of oppression]) . . . and (f) *postmodern and *deconstructive theory (. . . emphasis on discourse, narrative, and text) (pp. 217–226).

Feminist research may use *ethnographic, *grounded theory, *hermeneutic and *phenomenological research strategies as vehicles and frequently adopts a *critical theory stance; but there is much experimentation in feminist inquiries (often framed as *womanist* research by women of color scholars). Pressing issues faced by all researchers in this large field of studies are what the relationships of study participants to researchers and to research products are to be (the ethics of feminist research), how participants' *voices are to be heard, and how their stories are to be told (issues of *representation).

In the nursing literature, see a series of feminist grounded theory articles by Wuest (1995, 1998), Merritt-Gray and Wuest (1995), Wuest and Merritt-Gray (2001). See also J. Anderson et al. (2003), Fraser and Strang (2004), Georges (2002), Phillips and Drevdahl (2003), and J. Y. Taylor (2004).

Fieldnotes

Fieldnotes are written detailed descriptions of researchers' observations, experiences, and conversations in the 'field' (natural research setting). Fieldworkers produce them from 'jottings,' 'scratch notes,' or audio-taped self-recordings that serve as memory aids until there is an opportunity to produce a more comprehensive written account. A disciplined approach in writing up the fuller accounts soon after exiting the field maximizes the memory retention that is required in this activity. Style and format are researcher-determined; but there should be order and systemization as well as space allowances to insert codes and analytic notes over time. Descriptions of the researcher's personal insights and comments about field experiences need to be easily distinguishable from descriptions of the researcher's sense observations. Some field researchers keep a separate personal journal in which they record their thoughts, feelings, questions, hunches, and ideas. Sanjek's (1990) edited volume is a classic resource on the topic.

See **Fieldwork** and **Participant Observation.**

Fieldwork

In traditional ethnographic/anthropological research, *fieldwork* involves prolonged residence with members of the culture that is being studied. Modified field approaches typically do not involve co-residence; but there is the expectation that the research will involve 'going to' research participants wherever they are. In nursing research 'the field' may be an emergency room, ICU, clinic, participants' private homes, or some combination thereof. Sometimes, instead of being a definite place or locale, 'the field' is a set of relationships with individuals whose common interests and experiences are associated with a research topic. However, fieldwork is not just about locating and gaining entry to the field. It is expected that time spent in the field will be sufficient to support the credibility of the research. Another expectation is that fieldwork will involve the combined research activities of *participant observation* and *in-depth interviews* that inform one another. Nevertheless, in many reports of ethnographic and other types of field research, background understandings obtained through participant observation are not evident because of heavy emphasis on the interview data. Sandelowski (2002) has raised concerns about privileging interviews in qualitative research to the neglect of other data categories. In field research it is the *triangulation of information sources that provides the quality of data necessary for accurate and insightful descriptions and interpretations.

See **Participant Observation.**

Focus Groups

Focus groups generate data on a designated topic through discussion and interaction. Participants are systematically selected on the basis of their ability to provide the most meaningful information on the topic. Sessions are moderated by a group leader and are conducted as informal semi-structured interviews. Often group interviews are used in conjunction with other forms of data collecting in larger quantitative or qualitative studies. When focus groups are used as the sole research strategy, they represent a distinct form of study with a history in marketing research. See Krueger and Casey (2000) for information on focus group techniques. For nursing research examples see P. McCarthy, Chammas, Wilimas, Alaoui, and Harif (2004), Salazar, Napolitano, Schere, and McCauley (2004) (including commentaries by R. A. P. Smith, 2004, and Daroszewski, 2004, and the authors' response), and Villarruel, Harlow, Lopez, and Sowers (2002).

Formal Theory

In qualitative theory-generating research, *formal theory* is at a higher level of abstraction and, therefore, more widely generalizable than context-specific *substantive theory*. However, substantive theory offers a starting point for the development of databased formal theory. Olshansky (1996) and Kearney (1998) discuss techniques for synthesizing findings from diverse studies of specific situations to generate formal theory in a broader substantive area. For example, Olshansky (1996, 2003) demonstrates a trajectory of theory development based on a series of linked studies in her research program on infertility and, subsequently, presents a theoretical perspective on the potential vulnerability to depression in previously infertile new mothers. See also Kearney's (2001a) synthesis of 13 qualitative research reports that produced a grounded formal theory of women's experience of domestic violence.

See **Substantive Theory.**

F

Frequency Distribution

A *frequency distribution* is a count of each of the different values for a variable. Most frequency distributions are 'univariate,' that is, for one variable at a time. But bivariate (and even multivariate) frequency distributions are of considerable interest as they provide counts for cross-tabulations of values that give some indication of the relationships between variables.

Perhaps the most important frequency distribution in the study of statistics is the theoretical 'normal,' or bell-shaped, distribution for which most of the values are in the center of the distribution and very few are located at the extremes. Other important frequency distributions are the t, F, and chi-square sampling distributions that are used in inferential statistics.

Frequency distributions are often characterized according to their degrees of 'skewness' and 'kurtosis.' A distribution that has several observations (a 'hump') at the low end of the scale and very few (a 'tail') at the high end of the scale is called *positively* skewed, or skewed to the right, whereas a distribution that is heavy at the high end and light at the low end is called *negatively* skewed, or skewed to the left. (See Norris & Aroian, 2004, for an interesting discussion of skewed distributions and their transformations.) A distribution that has an unusually large concentration of scores near the middle of the distribution is referred to as *leptokurtic;* if the distribution is 'flat' with approximately equal frequencies throughout the scale, it is called *platykurtic;* and the intermediate case is *mesokurtic.*

Example: A frequency distribution of the birth years (1946–1964) of the members of the baby boom cohort would provide the numbers of births for each of those years.

Functionalism

In the social sciences, *functionalism* (superceded by and sometimes used interchangeably with *structural-functionalism*) is a perspective on how components of social systems (e.g., customs and rituals or kinship/family, religious, political, and economic institutions) function to meet the needs of their members/society. It is based on the assumption of system stability (homeostasis), where change in one part will produce changes in all the others (interdependency). Major proponents of this way of thinking were: in anthropology—Bronislaw Malinowski (1884–1942) and A. R. Radcliffe-Brown (1881–1955); and, in sociology—Emile Durkheim (1858–1917) and Talcott Parsons (1902–1979). *Structural-functionalism* was the dominant perspective in sociology well into the 1970s. It was challenged on many fronts, including its assumptions about a positively purposeful, balanced interrelationship of parts to the whole, which failed to account for disharmony, conflict, and unintended consequences. Robert Merton's (1910–2003) work attempted to address some of these weaknesses. *Conflict theory* arose as a reaction against structural-functionalism. *Neofunctionalism* constituted an attempt to build on some of its stronger features. Although it is no longer a dominant sociological perspective, functionalism and structural-functionalism have been influential in shaping many of the theories (*borrowed and shared) that nurses use in education, practice, and research (e.g., adaptation, goal-attainment, role, and family systems theories).

G

Generalizations

Generalizations are inferences in the form of summary statements about the results of empirical, interpretive, or abstract theoretical investigations. In research, general principles are inferred from particular pieces of evidence. For example, in experimental research the statistical analysis of the data might suggest that the findings are so strong that they are *statistically* generalizable to other like cases that make up the larger population from which the study sample was drawn. Similarly, in qualitative research, interpretive analysis of the data might suggest that the findings are *theoretically* generalizable to other cases of similar type and circumstances. *Statistical generalizations* are *nomothetic,* which means that they are attempts to establish general, universal, lawlike principles based on probability (the likelihood that a particular event or relationship will occur). *Theoretical* or *analytical generalizations* are *idiographic,* which means that they are attempts to present knowledge based on specific cases in such a manner that it may be of service in resolving questions/issues in comparable cases. An example of how this works would be in the practice of case law.

See **Inference.**

Generalized Estimating Equations

Generalized estimating equations (GEE) are methods that are used, primarily in epidemiological research, for analyzing data for persons nested within clusters, where the observations within cluster are not independent of one another.

For technical details regarding this technique see Hanley, Negassa, Edwardes, and Forrester (2003) and/or J. W. Hardin and Hilbe (2003).

Grand Theory

See **Broad-Range Theory** and **Theory.**

Grounded Theory

Grounded theory is a qualitative research approach developed by Glaser and Strauss (1967) for the purpose of generating theory about how persons progress/move through life experiences. The theory remains connected to ('grounded in') the data in which it was generated through examples and explanations that show the fit between the theory and supporting empirical evidence. Progression/movement is described as a process expressed in terms of stages or phases (e.g., stages/phases of adjusting to a new situation, coping with illness or loss). The goal is to discover a core category that 'unlocks' the process through a *constant comparative method* of data analysis. This involves *coding data, creating and naming *categories, constantly comparing incoming *fieldwork data against already collected information, writing analytic notes (*memos/memoing), analyzing *negative cases, and using *theoretical sampling* to direct data gathering toward *saturation of categories (i.e., completeness). The core category, or *basic social process* (BSP), is the basis for theory generation. It recurs frequently, links all the data together, and illustrates the characteristic patterning of the experience, regardless of the various conditions under which it occurs and the different ways that people go through it. [Note: Some authors use BSP to stand for 'basic social problem' and identify the core variable as either a basic social psychological process (BSPP) or a basic social structural process (BSSP). Of the two, the term BSPP is more common.] *Substantive theory* that results from these analytic procedures allows for a deeper understanding of the human experience of interest to the researcher. (*Formal theory,* generally, is the result of the analysis of multiple substantive theories related to a topic.) *Symbolic interaction* is the theoretical perspective that guides grounded theory methodology. This is the view that human behavior is the result of basic social processes that can be understood by analyzing the nature of social interactions and the symbolic meanings conveyed by persons' actions in varying situations.

Differences between 'Straussian' and 'Glaserian' styles of grounded theory are the result of historical evolution of the method subsequent to the publishing of a text by Strauss and Corbin (1990) which Glaser (1992) believed was a distortion of original thinking about methods. Many of the differences relate to the addition of *axial coding* procedures, which involve use of a prescribed coding paradigm ('the conditional matrix') with predetermined subcategories intended to help researchers pose questions about the properties of and relationships in their data. Glaser (1978) argued that his examples of 18 different 'coding families' that may be used to systematically link categories of data illustrate but do not limit possibilities (i.e., they allow for 'emergence' of patterns versus 'forcing'). Alternative methods continue to emerge that

G

retain the ideas intrinsic to grounded theory but provide new frameworks for analytic processes, such as Schatzman's (1991) *dimensional analysis* model.

For examples of grounded theory research in the nursing literature, see Canales and Geller (2004), S. S. Kim (2004), Norton and Bowers (2001), and Perry (2002).

See **Symbolic Interaction.**

Guttman Scale

A set of test items is said to constitute a *Guttman scale* if the response to any item is perfectly predictable from the total test score.

The term derives from the psychologist Louis Guttman (1941), who first developed the concept. Because no set of actual test items exactly satisfies the defining property, it is common to talk about the extent to which a collection of items does constitute a perfect Guttman scale. A statistic called the coefficient of reproducibility measures that.

Example: A test of racial prejudice consisting of items such as "I would be willing to vote for a person of another race," "I would be willing to marry a person of another race," and so forth should approximate a Guttman scale and have a very high coefficient of reproducibility. Respondents might 'fall off the ladder' at different points of the scale, with some not even endorsing the former item, but anyone who endorses the latter item is almost certain to endorse the former item as well, so that there should be a very strong association between the *number* of items endorsed and *which* items are endorsed.

G

H

Halo Effect

Halo effect is the name given to the phenomenon whereby people, such as evaluators, tend to be influenced by their previous judgments of something, such as performance or personality. The name implies that a good impression at the outset will carry over into future evaluations regardless of differences in quality or character of presentation. However, the same tendency would apply to an initial negative impression—that is, a negative bias similarly might carry over into future evaluations.

Halo effect may be addressed by having evaluators complete an entire set of evaluations before moving on to the next and by concealing their previous responses as they move on to future evaluations.

See **Artifact.**

Hawthorne Effect

Hawthorne effect is the name given to the phenomenon whereby people who know that they are participants in a study are likely to behave differently from the way they would behave without that knowledge.

The name comes from one of the original industrial-psychological studies, carried out in the 1920s at the Hawthorne plant of the Western Electric Corporation in Cicero, Illinois. In that study, no matter what sorts of experimental treatments were tried out on the employees (raising the lighting, lowering the lighting; raising the temperature, lowering the temperature; and other interventions) their productivity went up. The only explanation that could be provided at the time was that the employees were so grateful for the special attention that they tried to please the investigators in the best way they knew how, that is, by increased productivity.

The Hawthorne effect can also work in reverse. People can be so upset about being studied that they perform *worse* than they otherwise might.

There are two 'cures' for the Hawthorne effect. The first, and better of the two, is to randomly assign subjects to experimental and control groups who *all* know that they are being studied; if the experimental group 'wins' it will be an effect over and above the Hawthorne effect. The second is to carry out research on human beings totally without their knowledge, so that the Hawthorne effect has no opportunity to manifest itself. Such an approach raises some serious ethical problems, however.

Example: In an experimental study of the relative effects of visual stimuli and audial stimuli on reaction time, participating subjects should be told that they will be receiving one type of stimulus or the other, but they should not be told which one they will get. The Hawthorne effect may operate, but it should be 'balanced' across the two groups.

See **Artifact.**

Health Services Research (HSR)

The Institute of Medicine defines *health services research (HSR)* as "a multidisciplinary field of inquiry, both basic and applied, that examines the use, costs, quality, accessibility, delivery, organization, financing, and outcomes of health care services for individuals and populations" (Field, Tranquada, & Feasley, 1995, p. 3). HSR draws on many academic and professional fields (e.g., epidemiology, economics, nursing, medicine, biostatistics), utilizing a variety of techniques from descriptive observational epidemiology to intervention trials/clinical research, and it places more emphasis on feasibility testing (e.g., population-based interventions or programs) versus theory testing. Thus, within the spectrum of research it is usually more focused on actual 'real world' application than the validity of interventions under 'ideal' circumstances. The hallmark of HSR is addressing three key components of health care services . . . structure, processes, and outcomes. For example, Harrington, Woolhandler, Mullan, Carrillo, and Himmelstein (2001) address structural aspects of nursing home care—nursing home ownership and level of nurse staffing—as they relate to health outcomes. N. M. Watson, Brink, Zimmer, and Mayer (2003) address the occurrence of clinical problems, specifically, the incidence of incontinence in nursing homes, and the processes used to evaluate and treat them. And, Bates-Jensen et al. (2003) address how processes (actual care) relate to health outcomes (pressure ulcers).

Terms closely related to HSR include *outcomes research* and *evaluation research.* According to the Agency for Healthcare Research and Quality (AHRQ) "outcomes research . . . evaluates the impact of health care on health outcomes of patients and populations" (Stryer, Siegel, & Rodgers, 2004, p. III-1). Thus, *outcomes research,* defined in this way, is clearly a subset of *health services research* even though the term 'outcomes research' is used in other ways. There also is a certain lack of clarity in

H

73

the ways that the terms *health services research* and *evaluation research* are used. In this dictionary, we subsume *quality assurance/continuous quality improvement* activities under evaluation research. However, there is considerable overlap between evaluation research and health services research. Finally, see also Jennings (2004) for a helpful discussion of the definitional boundaries between *health services research (HSR)* and *nursing administration research (NAR)* (which she describes as a subset of HSR).

See **Evaluation Research** and **Outcomes Research.**

Hermeneutic Circle

The idea of *the hermeneutic circle* refers to the nature and process of textual understanding that unites the interpreter and the work (a text or experience) that is to be interpreted. Linguistically, the circle represents the mental process, i.e., conversational or *dialectical* interaction that occurs as an interpretation unfolds with the whole (entire text) and the parts (individual concepts) constantly informing one another. The image is one of the *parts* that form the circle, the circle as a *whole* that defines the parts (both in constant interaction) and the *meaning* that stands *within* the hermeneutic circle. Logically, the interpretive act involves a mental *leap into* the circle that enables a grasp of the whole and the parts together. As a spatial image, the circle represents an area of *shared understanding* between the text's author and the interpreter; and its shape represents ongoing dialogue. That is, conversation never leaves the hermeneutic circle because interpretations cannot be verified. They lead to further interpretations that engage with previous ones and enter into their own **dialectic* between the parts and the whole.

See **Hermeneutics.**

Hermeneutics

Historically, *hermeneutics* (a word derived from Hermes, who served the other Greek Gods as a bearer of messages to mortals) was concerned with the interpretation of Biblical texts. The original focus was on recovering the authentic versions of scriptures that were prone to numerous errors from hand copying prior to the age of the printing press. However, early in the 19th century, interest turned to issues of how to interpret any text, not only by fixing attention on the work itself but also by taking into consideration the experiences of its author. Reconstruction of the meanings that a writer has intended to convey implies a relationship between reader and text that is like a conversation or **dialectic*. The philosopher Dilthey (1833–1911) saw the text as *lived experience* that can be understood by readers who try to imaginatively put themselves in the position of the text's creator. For Gadamer (1900–2002), hermeneutic

H

understanding involves creating a relationship between the linguistic and historic context of the interpreter and of the text to be interpreted and understood. This represents *the hermeneutic circle,* i.e., the possibility of achieving understanding that is always tentative, forever ongoing, and subject to revision. Ricoeur (1913–) extended the idea of hermeneutics as textual analysis to any human situation, which then is to be *read* (i.e., interpreted) as a text. Ricoeur also introduced the importance of *the hermeneutics of suspicion* as well as *the hermeneutics of affirmation,* thus introducing the idea of *critical hermeneutics.* *Critical hermeneutics denies that there is an escape from unavoidable biases introduced by such conditions as class, race, and gender. Therefore, the objective of critical hermeneutics is to reveal or *unmask* false consciousness by calling it into awareness.

Hierarchical Linear Modeling

Hierarchical Linear Modeling (HLM) is a type of statistical analysis in which the data are analyzed both for individual subjects within one or more aggregates and for the aggregates themselves. Each is called a 'level' of analysis (not to be confused with a 'level' of measurement). In the older literature such an approach was typically subsumed under the heading of 'unit of analysis problems' (see the unit of analysis entry).

In a methodological article, Cho (2003) provided a good discussion of HLM and in a subsequent article Cho, Ketefian, Barkauskas, and Smith (2003) reported the use of HLM in their study of nurse staffing. See also Wu (1995) and Raudenbush and Bryk (2002).

Hierarchical Regression Analysis

Hierarchical regression analysis is a type of regression analysis in which the independent variables are 'entered' sequentially into the analysis in accordance with some theoretical model. It tests the 'effect' of one or more variables over and above other variables. Koniak-Griffin, Lesser, Uman, and Nyamathi (2003) used hierarchical regression analysis in their study of unprotected sexual activity among teenagers.

HIPAA

In the United States, the *Health Insurance Portability and Accountability Act* (better known as *HIPAA*) is a first-time enactment into law (effective April 14, 2003) of nationwide privacy and security standards developed by the Department of Health and Human Services and designed to protect individuals' medical records and other identifiable health information (on paper, in computers, or communicated orally). The *HIPAA privacy rule* establishes standards to protect the *confidentiality of individually identifiable health information, granting new rights to individuals regarding protected health information about them and mandating compliance from health care providers, health plans, and health care clearinghouses. The *HIPAA security rule* sets standards for the security of protected health information that is collected, maintained, used, or transmitted electronically, requiring that measures be taken to secure this information while in the custody of entities 'covered' by HIPAA (health care plans, providers, or clearinghouses) as well as while in transit between covered entities and from covered entities to others. HIPAA's impact on research is related to the privacy and security regulations governing *protected health information (PHI)* and all procedures necessary to assure compliance with these federally mandated regulations.

See **Protected Health Information.**

Historical Research

Historical research involves the systematic investigation and critical review of past events for the purposes of setting the record straight, discovering links with the past that explain or increase understanding of present events and circumstances, and answering questions about developments and trends. "In contrast to nostalgia, history attempts to recapture the complex ways that the persons and ideas of the past have influenced the present" (Hamilton, 1993, p. 48).

Historical inquiry involves intensive searches for, and concentrated analysis of, existing literature, documents, artifacts, photographs, and recordings on the phenomenon of interest. Oral histories, involving interviews with persons who are knowledgeable about historical events or personages, provide another type of information that broadens the range of data collection significantly. They allow for more creativity on the part of the researcher, who typically in historical research has no control over the quantity or the quality of data. With living sources of data, joint probing, searching, and reflecting on the targeted themes and questions may lead to rewarding and unexpected insights.

Sources of historical data are designated as primary sources (original documents, memorabilia, firsthand accounts) or secondary sources (summaries and interpretations of primary source material by other persons). Primary sources are of greater value because the potential for distortion or bias beyond the researcher's control is reduced. Historical data are evaluated for authenticity and estimated value, in terms of accuracy.

The historiographer addresses research questions and/or tests hypotheses, sometimes statistically, but more often by logical interpretation of relationships among phenomena of interest suggested by the amassed data. Qualitative methods of data analysis may be used to arrive at inferences about hypothesized relationships. These involve identification of themes or patterns in the data that guide the interpretation.

H

The American Association for the History of Nursing (AAHN) has published a position paper, based on the work of Keeling and Ramos (1995), advocating the inclusion of nursing history in the curricula of all undergraduate and graduate nursing programs. It recommends, for doctoral level students, inclusion of content on sound historical research methods. The rationale, in part, states:

> Nurses in the 21st century will need more than sheer information; they will need a greater sensitivity to contextual variables and ambiguity if they are to critically evaluate the information they receive. . . . History offers not only contextual perspective, but also enlightenment. . . . Nursing history . . . serves to expand students' thinking and provides them with a sense of professional heritage and identity . . . [and] knowledge of historical research methods broadens the repertoire of research skills of the graduate student (AAHN, 2001, pp. 1–2).

In the nursing literature, see Brush and Capezuti (2001), Brush et al. (1999), Connolly (2004), Fairman and Kagan (1999), Fealy (2004), Houweling (2004), Meehan (2003), Melchior (2004), Pfeil (2003), Porter and Bean (2004), and K. K. Thomas (2004).

See **Oral History.**

Holism

Holism is the idea that a phenomenon cannot be understood or explained by the sum of its parts. In systems thinking, holistic concepts are used to classify hierarchies of 'wholes' believed to be constituent parts of larger entities (e.g., quarks, protons, atoms, molecules, etc., in nature), the explanation of which cannot be understood solely on the basis of how their parts interact with one another. In theology and philosophy, holistic thinking holds that phenomena such as mind, soul, human life, and consciousness cannot be explained or grasped by the study of cells or body systems. Beliefs about holistic nursing practice stress the importance of using multiple approaches to understand the complex natures of individuals, groups, and communities. (See the entry on *patterns of knowing*.) Research methodologies also have been described as holistic (qualitative) and reductionistic (quantitative). However, for qualitative researchers the distinction has a lot to do with values and emphases placed on understanding phenomena in context.

See **Reductionism** and **Contextualism.**

Human Science

Human science, defined broadly, distinguishes between natural science disciplines and others focused more directly on problems of human existence. Specifically, the term is associated with a central theme of Wilhelm Dilthey's (1833–1911) philosophy of life, based on examination of human

H

and social studies *(Geisteswissenschaften)*. His interest was in the relationship between lived experience and an understanding *(Verstehen)* of how the mind directs and reveals itself in history and literature. Today the term is used to describe the focus of interpretivists who draw upon practices derived from a wide set of disciplines such as anthropology, history, literary criticism, philosophy, psychology, and sociology. A human science focus is concerned with interpreting the meaning of life experiences, in contrast to a natural science focus on providing causal explanations for them. It is based on the assumption that nature can be explained, but humans need to be understood. Phenomenologist van Manen (1990) relates human science inquiry to a study of meaning (patterns/structures/levels of experience); and nurse scientist Jean Watson (1985) relates a human science context to "a perspective that does not disengage nursing's ultimate meanings from its esthetics, ethics, science, and practice" (p. 16).

See **Phenomenology, Hermeneutics,** and **Patterns of Knowing.**

Hypothesis

In the context of a scientific theory, a *hypothesis* is a statement that usually postulates some sort of relationship between constructs (theoretical hypothesis) or variables (operational hypothesis) acknowledged to be crucial to that theory. In the more restrictive context of inferential statistics, a hypothesis is a conjecture regarding the numerical value of a population parameter. The two meanings have a great deal in common, however, as inferential statistics often plays a central role in the testing of scientific theory.

Example: ". . . we hypothesized that greater religiosity (religious practice, application, social support, identity, and commitment) is related to lower body weight, with psychosocial and health behaviors as mediators" (Kim, K. H., Sobal, & Wethington, 2003, p. 470).

Distinctions are typically drawn among hypotheses, propositions, axioms, and assumptions. Similarly, authors make distinctions among different kinds of hypotheses. For example, Polit and Beck (2004) discuss deductive versus inductive hypotheses, multivariate versus univariate hypotheses, simple versus complex hypotheses, and so on.

In traditional statistical hypothesis-testing, a so-called 'null' hypothesis is pitted against an 'alternative' hypothesis. The null hypothesis is usually a conjecture regarding *no* relationship, *no* difference, etc., that the investigator is inclined to disbelieve; the alternative hypothesis is often a research hypothesis that arises from some theory that the investigator is inclined to believe. Sample data are collected and a decision is made to reject or not reject the null hypothesis (one doesn't 'prove' or 'disprove' either hypothesis). The theory is thus strengthened, weakened, or modified.

H

The alternative hypothesis may be *directional* (e.g., the correlation between height and weight is greater than zero) or *nondirectional* (e.g., the correlation between height and weight is not equal to zero). The first example postulates a directional difference from zero, whereas the second example is the simple denial of the null hypothesis.

Example: 'Anxiety reduces achievement' is an example of an alternative research hypothesis that might be part of a theory of anxiety. To test that hypothesis one would actually determine whether or not its null counterpart, 'There is no relationship between anxiety and achievement,' can be rejected.

See **Theory** and **Proposition**.

Hypothesis Testing

Hypothesis testing has both a general scientific meaning and a specific statistical meaning. Any study that tests one or more tenets of a theory is referred to as hypothesis-testing. In addition, any study that employs a test of statistical significance is said to be using the hypothesis-testing form of statistical inference. The results either support or do not support the theory.

Hypothetico-Deductive Method

Hypothetico-deductive method is the covering-law model of scientific explanation that relies on theoretical explanation of a phenomenon (hypothesis formation) and experimentation (hypothesis testing).

See **Experiment** and **Explanation**.

H

I

Idealism

Idealism is the ontological assumption that there is no direct access to the external material world except through the mind. That is, the nature of being/reality rests with consciousness or reason. It opposes *realism,* which views the material world as 'objects' existing independent of human knowledge and awareness. There are a variety of idealist philosophies. In philosophy of science, the major ontological debates have been between realists and idealists. However, *anti-realism* is another position that more recently has entered into these dialogues.

See **Ontology** and **Realism.**

Ideology

An *ideology* is a set of beliefs based on core values, often directed toward political or social action in response to perceived oppression and domination. Creswell (1998) discusses three ideological perspectives (postmodernism, critical theory, and feminist approaches) that "draw attention to the needs of people and social action" (p. 78). When used in research, they guide choices about what to study and how to gather and analyze data. Crotty (1998) describes these three ideologies as theoretical perspectives.

See **Theoretical Perspective.**

Idiographic

Idiographic analysis is concerned with the particulars or unique aspects of persons, events, or cases that cannot be repeated. *Idiographic generalizations* are restricted to the specific case/circumstance and those thought to resemble it.

See **Case Study** and **Generalizations.**

Imputation

Imputation is one of the two principal ways of coping with missing-data problems (the other is deletion). Rather than deleting a 'case' from further analysis if it has any missing data, one or more estimates of the missing data are computed and the 'case' remains in the analysis.

For the same example considered in conjunction with the entry for *deletion,* if a particular respondent to a survey omitted just one of 100 items in that survey, the response (s)he 'might have made' could be estimated using the data for all of the other respondents and/or using the non-missing data for that subject. The simplest (albeit not the only and usually not the best) strategy is to assign to that non-respondent the mean of the 'scores' for the other subjects who did respond to the item. (One of the arguments against that strategy is that it artificially reduces the variance for that item, since the non-respondent's deviation from the mean is set equal to zero. For just one non-respondent and just one item the effect should be minimal, however.) There are several 'fancier' imputation methods, the most widely used strategies being the so-called 'Expectation Maximization (EM)' method and the multiple imputation methods advocated by Little and Rubin (2002) and others.

See **Deletion** and **Missing Data.**

Independent Observations

The observations ('pieces of data') in a research investigation are said to be independent if the measurement obtained on each subject neither influences nor is influenced by the measurement obtained on another subject.

The assumption of *independent observations* is crucial for all inferential statistical procedures but is often violated, especially in the application of chi-square to contingency tables. In such applications it is not uncommon to find that one or more persons have been counted in the data more than once. Whenever the number of observations is greater than the sample size there is a dependence-of-observations problem.

Example: In a study of the relationship between height and weight, Mary's height should be independent of Sally's height, unless they happen to be twins of one another. (Their weights are more likely to be more independent than their heights *even if* they are twins of one another.)

Independent Samples

Two or more samples are called independent if they are not matched with one another in any way.

Independent samples are very common in experiments; one sample is given the experimental treatment and the other sample is given the control treatment. They are also common in nonexperimental research concerned with sex differences, religious differences, and so forth.

Example: A cross-sectional study of the differences between 60-year-olds and 70-year-olds at a given point in time is likely to be based on independent samples (comparing a random sample of 200 60-year-olds with a random sample of 200 70-year-olds, say), whereas a longitudinal study of the differences between 60-year-olds and 70-year-olds must by definition use dependent samples (60-year-olds 'matched' with themselves when they are 70-year-olds 10 years later).

Independent Variable

An *independent variable* is a variable that is a potential cause of a dependent variable.

In an experiment an independent variable is actually 'manipulated;' that is, the investigator intervenes in the natural course of events and 'creates' a variable of two or more treatment conditions. In nonexperimental research an independent variable is merely measured and correlated with a dependent variable.

Example: In testing the 'effect' of stress on depression, where stress is the independent variable and depression is the dependent variable, one researcher might carry out an experiment by randomly assigning subjects to one of two stressful conditions and observing what happens to depression, but another researcher might measure stress, measure depression, and correlate the two.

Inductive Reasoning

Inductive reasoning is a way of thinking (a logical mental process) that begins with observation of patterns or repetitive occurrences and systematically formulates conclusions about what probably or possibly is going on, that is, what those observations may signify. Thus, conclusions are reached by moving from lower to higher levels of abstraction. In contrast, in deductive reasoning, conclusions are reached by moving in the opposite direction (higher to lower), beginning with a theory about what is going on and applying it to various propositions (e.g., through hypothesis-testing). Inductive methods are common in qualitative research where data analysis is an iterative process that also involves reflection, intuition, and introspection. It should be understood, however, that although research designs may be strongly associated with a certain style of reasoning, it is impossible to conduct any sort of scientific inquiry without the use of both approaches.

See **Deductive Reasoning** and **Theory.**

Inference

An *inference* is the act or process of using a statement, set of assumptions, proposition, or generalization as the basis for reaching a conclusion about something. Inferences systematically follow a logical path of reasoning that may be *deductive* (inferences in which the conclusion follows necessarily from the premises), *inductive,* (inferences in which the conclusion is based on specific observations or patterns), or *abductive* (inferences based on the best explanation of available data, i.e., hypothesizing). To *imply* (to suggest) is not the same as to *infer* (to explain) via statistical inference or narrative argument.

See **Generalizations** and **Explanation.**

Inferential Statistics

Inferential statistics is the branch of statistics that is concerned with procedures for making generalizations from samples to populations.

Populations are usually very large and not completely accessible, and it is often too expensive to study *all* of the members of a population. Therefore, the researcher typically draws a sample from the population (ideally at random), studies the sample in *its* entirety, and makes some sort of generalization from the sample to the population. Such generalizations are always subject to error (the smaller the sample the greater the expected error) unless the population is perfectly homogeneous with respect to the variable(s) of concern.

If one happens to have data for an entire population, there is no statistical inference to be made, but some researchers choose to "regard" certain small populations as samples from larger populations (see Barhyte, Redman, & Neill, 1990).

Inferential statistical procedures are of two types: (a) those concerned with the estimation of population parameters and (b) those concerned with the testing of hypotheses about population parameters. The latter procedures are far more common.

Subsumed under estimation are point estimation, in which the researcher gives a 'best guess' as to the actual value of a parameter based on the calculated value for the corresponding sample statistic, and interval estimation, in which a 'confidence interval' is established that has some specified degree of assurance for including the unknown value of the parameter. Point estimation is rarely employed, as it does not allow for any margin of error due to variability from sample to sample. Interval estimation is used quite often in survey research and in educational and psychological testing.

Rightly or wrongly, hypothesis testing gets 'all of the play' in research conducted in most of the social and biological sciences (including nursing). There are two types of hypothesis-testing procedures: (a) parametric tests, which make certain assumptions about the population(s); and (b) nonparametric tests, which do not make such assumptions.

Example: If the average age of a random sample of 200 Alzheimer's patients is found to be 73.8 years, it might be inferred that the average age of the population from which that sample was drawn is 73.8 *plus or minus* 3 years. And the hypothesis that the average age of Alzheimer's patients is 80 would be rejected.

I

The foregoing remarks regarding the principal kinds of inferential statistics, as well as the distinction between descriptive statistics and inferential statistics, can be summarized as follows:

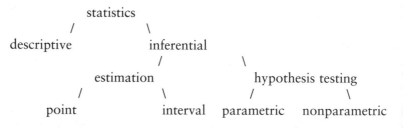

A particularly fine statistics textbook for nursing researchers is Munro (2001).

Informed Consent/Assent and Permission

Informed consent is the operationalization of the ethical principle of respect for persons. It involves a formal process that must be followed in the recruitment of potential research study subjects/participants. The three components of valid informed consent are: <u>information, understanding,</u> and <u>voluntary agreement</u> (Dunn & Chadwick, 2002, p. 99). The process is overseen by *Institutional Review Boards that must ensure that: (a) consent documents are clear, relevant, in language understandable to the potential subject (in plain English or in the language of the subject if English is not well understood), and contain all of the specific elements required by U.S. federal regulations; (b) persons obtaining consent have had ethics training and are knowledgeable about the study; (c) persons obtaining consent will not intentionally or unintentionally influence an individual's decision to participate in the research; (d) the timing and time allowed for the consent process will not impede an individual's ability to make a considered decision; and (e) the mode of presentation is appropriate and maximizes the individual's ability to make an informed choice about whether or not to participate in the research. In long, complex studies, renewal of consent may be required. There also are special conditions that are applicable to the protection of 'vulnerable subjects' as in the following examples.

<u>Vulnerable subjects</u>: "Because <u>children</u> cannot legally give consent, federal regulations require the *permission* of their parents, and with the exception of very young children in some treatment protocols, the *assent* (the affirmative agreement) of the child-subject" (Dunn & Chadwick, 2002, p. 103). State laws may apply to obtaining consent from <u>adults with limited capacity to consent</u>. Frequently employed techniques when enrolling these research subjects include: (a) *assent* (potential subject's affirmative agreement), (b) *permission* of legally authorized

representative/proxy, (c) staged consent, when subject's memory abilities are compromised, and (d) continuing evaluations of capacity and consent understanding (depending on the study). Special consideration also must be given to recruitment of institutionalized persons (e.g., in prisons, nursing homes, mental health facilities) involving extra steps to ensure that consent is voluntary, not coerced, and clear to individuals in terms of how the research will affect them. Other categories may be deemed as 'vulnerable' (e.g., pregnant women), depending on the nature of the research. Finally, although disenfranchised populations are not placed in the same category as 'vulnerable' subjects, Dunn and Chadwick offer good advice regarding the ethics of obtaining informed consent in these instances:

> The researcher must be clear about the intent of the research and the potential benefits to the community, if any. It is important not to overstate the potential benefits or promise resources that are not directly under the authority of the researcher. Communities that believe their participation will result in a guaranteed service that is not forthcoming will generally feel exploited. A good rule to follow is not to promise anything that you cannot guarantee (p. 112).

See Dunn and Chadwick's excellent manual on Protecting Study Volunteers in Research. Also see Crane and McSweeney (2004) on informed consent processes that facilitate older adults' participation in research and Mueller's (2004) ethnographic field study of the informed consent process and HIV/AIDS clinical trial work.

Institutional Review Board (IRB)

An *Institutional Review Board (IRB)* review and monitoring system is a U.S. federally mandated protective mechanism to ensure an independent ethical review of all proposed and ongoing research involving human subjects, as a condition set forth in institutional 'Assurances' filed with the government. The IRB has the authority to approve/disapprove, require modifications, continually monitor, re-approve, and terminate research activities as well as responsibilities to educate its members and investigators concerning the ethical conduct of research and to maintain comprehensive, detailed records in compliance with federal regulations. Violation of the obligations of an Assurance (e.g., a researcher's non-compliance with IRB requirements) can result in termination or suspension of the institution's Assurance, suspension or restrictions to all ongoing studies at the institution, disqualification of the institution and/or IRB from conducting and approving clinical research, and departmental and/or individual restrictions and sanctions (Dunn & Chadwick, 2002, pp. 36–43).

I

Instrumentation

Instrumentation is synonymous with measurement and is the term that is likely to be preferred in biophysiological research involving measuring devices actually constructed for some very specific purpose. The term is also preferred when identifying the data collection phase of a research design.

See **Design** and **Measurement.**

Intensive (In-Depth) Interviewing

Intensive (in-depth) interviewing involves use of open-ended <u>and</u> semi-structured interview guide formats with a conversational style that allows the interviewer to probe for underlying emotions, thoughts, and meanings. Qualitative researchers often use this technique. They prepare for an interview in advance by reviewing the primary questions the research is designed to answer, the specific questions they want to be sure to ask study participants, and the linkages between the two. Interviews tend to be long (up to 2 hours or more) and may be tape-recorded. However, this does not relieve the researcher from listening carefully to what the interviewee is saying and picking up on verbal and non-verbal cues that will help him/her to appropriately structure and maintain the interview content and climate. Interview transcripts will not contain all of the information the researcher needs to obtain from an in-depth interview, and they are vulnerable to errors. Therefore, it is important to listen, remember, and observe carefully in order to be able to supplement transcriptions with detailed *fieldnotes.

See **Transcription.**

Intent to Treat (Intention to Treat)

One of the terms that is often encountered in the evidence-based-practice (EBP) nursing literature is the concept of *intent to treat*. It arises in conjunction with a clinical trial (see entry for that term) in which subjects have been randomly assigned to treatment and control conditions, but some of the subjects do not participate in the condition to which they had been assigned or participate only in a limited extent. The problem is that the treatment and control groups are comparable at the point of assignment, and the decision by any subject to withdraw from the assigned condition could destroy that balance.

What is one to do if this should happen? The intent-to-treat strategy is to associate any data for a subject with the group (treatment or control) to which the subject had initially been assigned, even if that subject 'winds up' in the opposite group or has withdrawn from the study.

That sounds rather strange, particularly if one or more subjects actually receive the opposite treatment to which they were initially assigned and they're included in the data for the initial treatment. The rationale for doing so, however, is twofold: (1) if the objective of the study is to contribute to a 'real world' health care policy regarding two treatments for which total compliance is not possible, the principal concern is what treatment to recommend, not what treatment to scrutinize; and (2) the usual effect of an intent-to-treat analysis is conservative (the experimental treatment is at least that good) since most of the attrition takes place within the experimental treatment by subjects whose data, when included for that treatment, usually dampen its effect.

Long, Ritter, and Gonzalez (2003) used an intent-to-treat analysis in their randomized clinical trial of disease self-management.

See **Clinical Trial.**

Intentionality

Intentionality is a concept that defines the nature of consciousness by describing its relationship to the external world. It means that all thought is directed toward something (the *intentional object*), a distinguishing characteristic of psychic phenomena that is of major interest to phenomenologists.

See **Phenomenology.**

Interaction Effect

An *interaction effect* is a special kind of 'combination' effect of two or more independent variables on a dependent variable.

It is an effect that is different from a simple summarization of the effects of each of the independent variables taken separately. The term is usually associated with experimental research where a 'sex-by-treatment' interaction, for instance, may be of interest. The following example attests to other uses.

Example: If nurses have a life expectancy of 5 years above average, and researchers have a life expectancy of 3 years above average, one would expect that nurse researchers would have a life expectancy of 8 years above average. If they have a life expectancy either greater than or less than 8 years above average, then there is an interaction effect of the two independent variables (occupation and specialization) on the dependent variable (life expectancy).

Internal Consistency

Internal consistency is a type of reliability that is concerned with the extent to which the parts of a multi-item instrument 'hang together.' The most common procedures for determining the internal consistency of a measuring instrument are coefficient alpha (Cronbach's alpha) and split halves.

See **Coefficient Alpha, Reliability,** and **Split Halves.**

I

Internal Validity

Internal validity is a term that is synonymous with control. It was coined by Campbell and Stanley (1966). A design (usually an experimental design) is said to be internally valid if the effect alleged to be produced by the independent variable can actually be attributed to that variable and not to some competing 'threat' with which it is confounded.

As is the case with its companion term, external validity (generalizability), it is unfortunate that the term has the root word *validity,* because that is a measurement characteristic and not a design characteristic.

Example: A true experiment in which the subjects are randomly assigned to different drug treatments has very strong internal validity because the randomization process controls most variables that might otherwise be competing causes.

Lincoln and Guba (1985) have described *credibility* as a parallel to *internal validity* in qualitative research. Credibility is demonstrated by accuracy and validity of findings that are assured through multiple methods and careful documentation.

See **Trustworthiness Criteria.**

Internet Research

Internet research is a general term that is applied to any research in which the data are obtained using the World Wide Web (www). The advantage of such research is that very large numbers of potential research participants are accessible. For example, see AbuAlRub's (2004) Web-based hospital staff nurse survey. The principal disadvantages are that instruments employed in obtaining the data may not be as valid and reliable as they would be in more traditional settings, and the sample upon which the research is based may not be representative of the population to which one might want to generalize. A recent issue of *Advances in Nursing Science* (Vol. 26, No. 4, 2003) was devoted entirely to this topic, and two of the articles (LaCoursiere, 2003; Strickland et al., 2003) specifically addressed those disadvantages. The Strickland et al. article also contains a summary of a study (of migraine headaches in perimenopausal women) that was carried out on the Internet.

A serious issue related to Internet research is that "[t]he Web provides enormous potential for the invasion of privacy" (Cotton, 2003, p. 315). While secure Web sites are used for many kinds of health research, questions remain for researchers and Institutional Review Boards with regard to what may be considered as 'public behavior.' For example, is it ethical for a researcher to collect and analyze information from chat room support groups that may be freely accessed by the public without disclosing his/her presence and obtaining assent from participants? Or is it ethical for a researcher to pose as a participant in order to comment and ask questions that generate data? Although one might say that this is indeed unethical, "there is no one governing authority over the global medium of the Internet . . . to protect online users . . . [and a paucity of] *Institutional Review Board . . . guidelines for evaluating ethical risks and safeguards for research on the Internet" (Cotton, pp. 315–316).

See **Unobtrusive Research.**

Interpretation

In scientific inquiry, the term *interpretation* is used in two ways. In its most general sense, it applies to any explanation of the meaning of a phenomenon regardless of how that explanation was derived. In another sense, it is used to distinguish between interpretivist approaches to explanation and causal, lawlike explanatory models.

See **Explanation, Interpretivism,** and **Thick Description.**

Interpretivism

Interpretivism is a theoretical perspective/paradigm that informs several research methodologies (e.g., interpretive ethnography, grounded theory, phenomenological and hermeneutic research) whose general aim is to provide "culturally derived and historically situated interpretations of the social life-world" (Crotty, 1998, p. 67). The intellectual roots of interpretive research approaches (called *the interpretive turn*) can be traced back to philosopher Dilthey's (1833–1911) rejection of empiricism and the efforts of sociologists Weber (1864–1920) and Schutz (1899–1959) to define the work of their discipline in terms of *Verstehen* (*understanding* in German) as that applies to the subjective meanings that people give to their actions. However, Weber viewed *Verstehen* as being contributory and preliminary to methods of causal explanations of human behavior. Consequently, "while continuing to trace its lineage back to Weber . . . the *Verstehen* approach has not maintained his passion for empirical verification or his concern to explain in causal terms" (Crotty, p. 71).

In response to positivist criticisms of interpretivism as an unverifiable, naïve attempt to *get inside the heads* of subjects, philosopher Charles Taylor (1931–), anthropologist Clifford Geertz (1923–), and others have attempted to clarify how the dialogic methodologies of *Verstehen* approaches to human inquiry involve something more and different than psychological closeness or empathy. As Geertz (1983b) explains:

> The trick is not to get yourself into some inner correspondence of spirit with your informants. Preferring like the rest of us to call their souls their own, they are not going to be altogether keen about such an effort anyhow. The trick is to figure out what the devil they think they are up to. . . . Whatever accurate to half-accurate sense one gets of one's informants are, as the phrase goes, really like . . . comes from the ability to construe their modes of expression, what I would call their symbol systems (pp. 58, 70).

Thus, the focus is on producing explanations that do not serve the same purposes and are not like causal, lawlike theoretical explanations of human actions. (See Crotty, 1998, and Schwandt, 2000, for descriptions of different understandings of *Verstehen* approaches.)

The interpretive turn initiated an ongoing dialogue about the *deconstruction of the *positivist and *postpositivist idea of science and marked an increasing use of interpretive approaches in the social/human sciences (see Rabinow & Sullivan, 1979, & Schwandt, 2000). *Hermeneutics, *phenomenology, and *symbolic interaction are theoretical perspectives that fall under the broad umbrella of interpretivism.

See **Explanation** and **Interpretation.**

Inter-Rater Reliability

Inter-rater reliability is a type of reliability that involves an assessment of the extent to which two or more raters (scorers, judges) agree regarding the ratings (scores, judgments) they give to the behaviors they observe. The term is synonymous with *objectivity* in this context.

See **Reliability.**

Intersubjectivity

Intersubjectivity is a concept that concerns subjective interpretations of experience that are accessible to more than one individual (i.e., shared or common interpretations or perceptions). The creation of meaning through the interplay of individual subjectivities is a natural characteristic of the *lifeworld* that is of interest to phenomenologists and other interpretivists. (The term is used in other contexts as well, particularly where there is disagreement. For example, *intersubjectivity* might indicate a *consensus* regarding the *objectivity* of a particular phenomenon or research finding.)

See **Phenomenology.**

Interval Estimation

Interval estimation is a type of statistical inference in which a 'confidence interval' is constructed around an obtained sample statistic in such a manner that it has some specified degree of assurance for including the corresponding population parameter.

See **Inferential Statistics.**

Interval Scale

An *interval scale* is a level of scientific measurement characterized by the existence of a constant unit of measurement and an arbitrary zero point. The only permissible transformations of interval scales are those of the linear form $Y = a + bX$.

Example: Temperature measured on the centigrade (Celsius) scale is an interval scale, because the centigrade degree is constant throughout the scale, the zero point is arbitrary (the point at which water becomes ice), and the only permissible transformations are transformations such as the change from centigrade (C) to Fahrenheit (F) by the equation F = 32 + 1.8C.

See **Scale.**

Intervening Variable

An *intervening variable* is a variable that is in between an independent variable and a dependent variable in a causal sequence, and can therefore produce an *indirect* effect of the independent variable on the dependent variable in addition to, or instead of, a direct effect.

Effect: Anxiety can have both a direct effect on achievement and an indirect effect on achievement through the intervening variable of (lack of) motivation.

Intraclass Correlation

Intraclass correlation is a type of correlation usually associated with inter-rater reliability, but it can be applied to other correlational situations. The key difference between intraclass correlation and traditional Pearson product-moment correlation (which is sometimes called interclass correlation) is that in intraclass correlation the variances of the two variables being correlated must be equal or approximately equal. (There is no such restriction for Pearson r.)

In applications to inter-rater reliability, one actually can obtain two intraclass correlations: one for the average reliability of a single rater, and one for the reliability of the sum of the raters. It is the latter correlation that is of greater relevance, since the data are typically 'pooled' across raters.

Yen and Lo (2002) provide a good discussion of the application of intraclass correlation to test-retest reliability.

See **Reliability.**

I

K

Key Informant

A *key informant* is a person who can provide detailed or specialized information about his or her own culture. In ethnographic field studies, key informants are select individuals who often assist the researcher in establishing rapport with others in the community, serve as chief interpreters, and provide instruction and guidance with regard to language and cultural norms. Therefore, only certain research participants, <u>not</u> all participants, will be identified as key informants.

See **Ethnography.**

Known-Groups Technique

The *known-groups technique* is a procedure associated with criterion-related validity (some authors subsume it under construct validity). To 'validate' a particular measuring instrument (e.g., a test of anxiety), an investigation is made of the extent to which a group of subjects known or assumed to possess a large amount of the trait being measured (e.g., anxiety) obtain scores on the instrument that are different from those obtained by a group of subjects known or assumed to possess a small amount of that trait.

An example of the use of the known-groups technique for instrument validation is provided by Creedy et al. (2003).

See **Validity.**

L

Law

A *law* is a proposition about the relationship between concepts in a theory that has been repeatedly supported and accepted as valid. Laws are highly generalizable; that is, they are consistently supported and not tentative. The social/human sciences have few laws in comparison to the physical sciences.

See **Theory** and **Proposition.**

Level of Significance

Level of significance, sometimes called significance level, is a term associated with the hypothesis-testing approach to statistical inference. It is the probability of rejecting a true null hypothesis, is usually denoted by the Greek letter alpha, and is conventionally set at .05, .01, or .001. For any given study, one and only one level of significance should be chosen, with all results interpreted with respect to that particular level (see Slakter, Wu, & Suzuki-Slakter, 1991).

See **Test of Significance.**

Life History

See **Biographical Method.**

Lifeworld/Lived Experience

In phenomenology, the *lifeworld (Lebenswelt),* or *lived experience,* is the natural world in which humans live. Because it consists of the commonsensical and that which is taken for granted, it tends to be less accessible. The goal of phenomenology is to return to this familiar world and re-examine through reflective awareness what human experiences are like from that vantage point. (There is a misleading tendency to use the term *lived experience* outside of its original context in place of other language to describe the focus of various other types of qualitative studies with an interest in human experience.)

See **Phenomenology.**

Likert Scale

A *Likert scale* is a type of test item in which respondents indicate their attitude toward a particular statement by choosing one of a small number of ordered alternatives.

The term is derived from the industrialist psychologist Rensis Likert (1932) who first used such scales. Most Likert scales consist of five scale points, usually designated by the words "strongly agree," "agree," "undecided," "disagree," and "strongly disagree." But there can be as few as two scale points or as many as 10 or more, and descriptors other than levels of agreement can also be used.

Example: In measuring attitudes toward abortion a researcher might present the statement "Abortion is murder" to a group of subjects and ask them to select one of the categories: "yes," "under certain circumstances," or "no" that best expresses their feelings regarding that statement.

See **Scale.**

LISREL

See **Structural Equation Modeling.**

Logical Empiricism

Logical empiricism is a theoretical perspective/paradigm that has informed contemporary mainstream philosophy of science definitions of standard *scientific method* (i.e., hypothetico-deductive method). Some see it as a more moderate version of *logical positivism*. Others use the two terms interchangeably (Crotty, 1998). The logical empiricist view (promoted in the philosophy of science literature by Carnap, Hempel, Nagel, and Reichenbach) is that scientific inquiry should be value-free and limited to the study of relationships between phenomena that are directly accessible to observation. Critics have called this perspective *the received view* (Suppe, 1977), which "in any discipline usually denotes a set of ideas that are not to be challenged, the philosophical equivalent of being engraved on stone" (Meleis, 1997, p. 80). Although, from the 1950s to the present, thinkers such as Kuhn, Toulmin, and Feyerabend have generally rejected logical empiricism (particularly, the notion that science is value-free), this perspective's basic ideas are a dominant influence in scientific discourse and are foundational to positivist research practice in the current postpositivist/postempiricist era.

See **Logical Positivism, Postempiricism,** and **Postpositivism.**

L

Logical Positivism

Logical positivism is a theoretical perspective/paradigm promoted by the *Vienna Circle* (a group of philosophers and scientists that met in Vienna in the 1920s and early 1930s). Drawing on the *strict empiricism* of Locke, Berkeley, and Hume and the *positivism* of Comte, the logical positivists aimed to bring the logic and technical precision of mathematical theory to scientific inquiry. Leading contributors to this work were Bertrand Russell (1872–1970) and Ludwig Wittgenstein (1889–1951). Central to its philosophy was a strong mistrust of and animosity toward metaphysics, ethics, aesthetics, and theology combined with the assertion that the only legitimate approach to knowledge was through logic and empirical research (i.e., direct observation and experimentation). The primary instrument for excluding metaphysical views, ethical and aesthetic values, and religious beliefs was the *verification principle* stipulating that no proposition may be considered meaningful (i.e., factual) unless verified through sense experience. Because propositions related to these other knowledge forms were deemed unverifiable by this approach, they were judged as perhaps "emotionally . . . or even spiritually of great value to people, but [unscientific and, therefore,] meaningless" (Crotty, 1998, p. 26). Logical positivism flourished for several decades before persistent criticism brought about its reintroduction in the somewhat more moderate guise of *logical empiricism*.

See **Empiricism Logical Empiricism, Positivism, Postempiricism,** and **Postpositivism.**

Logistic Regression Analysis

Logistic regression analysis is a special type of regression analysis in which the dependent variable is usually a dichotomy. (It has been extended to the situation where there are more than two categories for the dependent variable—see Kwak & Clayton-Matthews, 2002.)

Menard's (1995) monograph on logistic regression analysis is a very good 'how-to' source; and Zerwic, Ryan, DeVon, and Drell (2003) used logistic regression analysis in their study of differences in delaying treatment for acute myocardial infarction symptoms.

See **Regression Analysis.**

L

Longitudinal Study

A *longitudinal study* is a type of research in which one or more groups of people are studied at several points in time.

Longitudinal Study

Typical longitudinal research involves a single cohort (either an entire population or a sample therefrom) that is followed across time to investigate its development with respect to some dependent variable.

For an example of longitudinal research see the article by DiMattio and Tulman (2003) on the change in functional status of women who have undergone coronary artery bypass graft surgery.

L

M

Main Effect

Main effect is a term associated with the effect (causal or noncausal) on a dependent variable of a single independent variable considered separately from other independent variables.

The term is used most commonly in experimental research in which a factorial design assessing the effects of two or more independent variables has been used. The main effect of each independent variable is studied in conjunction with the combined (interaction) effects.

Example: The main effect of type of analgesic on reported pain is of considerable interest, in addition to the effect for males versus females, older people versus younger people, and the like.

Manipulation

Manipulation is the defining feature of an experiment. An investigation should be called an experiment if and only if the researcher directly 'manipulates' the independent variable, that is, actively intervenes to create some sorts of treatment conditions.

Sometimes it is difficult to determine whether or not the manipulation criterion has been satisfied. If some person other than the researcher intervenes and the researcher then studies the phenomenon, a case could be made that such a study also falls under the heading of an experiment, even though the administration of the experimental treatments has not been directly under the researcher's control.

Example: An investigator who is sincerely interested in the effect of sex education on the incidence of teenage pregnancies should directly manipulate the independent variable by assigning students (ideally at random) to receive or not receive sex education, rather than seek out, after the fact, one group of students who have been exposed to sex education and another group of students who have not been exposed to sex education.

See Experiment.

M

Matching

Matching is a technique sometimes used in experimental research in which each subject receiving the treatment is paired with another subject not receiving the treatment in an attempt to control for one or more characteristics that the paired subjects have in common. It is often, but mistakenly, believed that such a technique is superior to random allocation of subjects to treatment groups. (Campbell & Stanley, 1966, discuss the weaknesses of matching as an experimental research strategy.)

See **Control** and **Blocking.**

Mean

The *mean* (arithmetic mean) of a set of data for a variable is the sum of all the scores (the term *score* is used to refer to any numerical measurement) divided by the number of scores. It is the most commonly encountered statistic in nursing research because it is the traditional 'average' and researchers are often interested in the difference between the average scores on a particular variable for two or more groups of subjects, to determine the 'effect' (not necessarily in the causal sense) of group membership on that variable.

Measurement

The term *measurement* is usually associated with the operationalization of abstract constructs into concrete variables but can include anything from careful description to formal assignment of numbers to objects according to well-defined rules.

When careful description is the main concern, there may be less conscious thought of operationalization. However, the fact that decisions must be made about which empirical realities to observe and how they will be observed implies some sort of operationalization.

It is helpful to think about measurement as the process of translating some sort of reality into numbers. When a construct, for example, height is operationalized, each object to be measured is assigned a number. It may be very precise, for example, Mary is 68.7 inches tall; very rough, for example, Mary is a 1 (where 1 = tall, 0 = short, i.e., not tall); or anything in between.

The psychologist E. L. Thorndike (1918) once said: "Whatever exists at all exists in some amount" (p. 16). That claim was later followed up by the educator W. A. McCall (1939), who said: "Anything that exists in amount can be measured" (p. 18). To talk about something like height, sex, social support, or any other construct, it must be at least theoretically possible to measure it, and at least two different "scores" must be obtainable.

M

In quantitative studies, measurement considerations arise when attention is given to data collection. This is sometimes called the 'instrumentation' phase of the research, which comes between the overall design for the study and the analysis of the results. It is somewhat less important than the design phase, because unless the research problem is well thought out, good measures of various constructs won't help very much. But it is certainly much more important than the analysis phase, because meaningless measurements are not worth analyzing.

Example: The construct "Contraceptive Use" presents enormous measurement problems. First, is the focus to be on whether or not, which kind(s), how often, or just what? Second, how is the information to be obtained? Self-report? Probably, but such reports are subject to huge errors. Observation? Hardly, but that might be the most valid strategy. Third, who is (are) to be studied—only females who are involved in sexual activity? Only males? Both? If both, should *partners* be studied, given that contraception (or its lack) applies primarily to the act and not to separate individuals.

By way of contrast, "Spelling Ability" poses fewer problems. If you want to find out how much spelling ability a person has, you select a random sample of words from a dictionary and ask him or her to spell them.

Median

The *median* of a set of data for a variable is the middle value when the data are arranged from low to high (or high to low—it doesn't matter). The median is preferred to the mean when the variable being analyzed has a skewed frequency distribution and/or when the variable is ordinal rather than interval.

Mediating Variable

A *mediating variable* is the same as an intervening variable but usually carries the additional connotation of some sort of ameliorating or 'buffering' effect. People are always confusing the terms 'mediating variable' and 'moderator variable.' This is apparently because both mediating and moderator variables are third variables that play important roles in interpreting the relationship between two other variables. See Baron and Kenny (1986), Lindley and Walker (1993), and J. A. Bennett (2000) for excellent discussions of the difference between mediators and moderators; see J. A. Bennett, Stewart, Kayser, Jones, and Glaser (2002), Kearney, Munro, Kelly, and Hawkins (2004), Bruce, Lake, Eden, and Denney (2004), and Mahon, Yarcheski, and Yarcheski (2004) for nursing research examples, and see Dudley, Benuzillo, and Carrico (2004) for a discussion of computer programs that can be used for carrying out the analysis for mediating variables.

See **Buffering Variable, Intervening Variable,** and **Moderator Variable.**

M

Member Checks

In qualitative research, *member checks* involve ongoing informal and formal validation of data with study participants from whom the data were collected. Member checking is a way of establishing accuracy and overall credibility of the research. However, member checks can be problematic when researchers' findings uncover implicit patterns or meanings of which informants are unaware. Also, member checks are seldom useful in corroborating reports that are a synthesis/final interpretation of multiple perspectives, because individuals are not positioned well to account for perspectives beyond their own. Therefore it is up to the researcher to determine when and under what circumstances to use member checks (Morse, 1998a; Sandelowski, 1993).

Memos/Memoing

In qualitative research, analytic note writing (referred to as *memos/memoing* in *grounded theory) is an expected aspect of the research process. It occurs across the life of the research and is a record of the ideas that the researcher has about the nature of the data and how different concepts may be linked to one another. They are written into *fieldnotes and/or filed separately. However they are managed, analytic memos facilitate and keep track of theoretical thinking about the nature and content of the data and direction of the research.

See **Audit Trail.**

Meta-Analysis

A *meta-analysis* is a statistical amalgam of the findings of a number of research studies that have been carried out on a particular topic. It is sometimes referred to as an "analysis of analyses" (Glass, G. V, 1976), but it is really a *synthesis* (a bringing together of the analyses of separate investigations of the same general phenomenon) rather than an *analysis* (a breaking down). The original investigators have done the analyzing; the meta-analyst synthesizes the results of those analyses.

Although the term is somewhat grandiose—and the prefix *meta* does not always carry the same meaning—meta-analysis is currently very popular, despite the contentions of a number of people who argue that it is not a particular worthwhile activity (see, for example, Eysenck, 1978). It seems like an excellent idea to be able to quantify and integrate the findings of several studies, but the technical problems are occasionally insurmountable. Conversely, the strength of meta-analysis is seen as its ability to determine consistency of findings across a large number of studies; therefore, it is considered to be the strongest evidence from an evidence-based practice perspective.

M

There are a variety of ways of carrying out a meta-analysis. The most common way involves the determination of some sort of an average 'effect size' across studies (see Glass, 1976). Most procedures make a number of arguable assumptions, however, such as the independence of the studies and the comparability of the measurements for the study variables.

The term *meta-analysis* is sometimes confused with the term *secondary analysis* (for which this dictionary includes a separate entry). They are quite different activities. G. V Glass's (1976) article makes the distinction very clearly and also points out how both activities differ from the 'primary analysis' carried out by the original researcher(s).

Reynolds, Timmerman, Anderson, and Stevenson (1992) provide an excellent summary of meta-analysis and its advantages and disadvantages. See also Conn and Rantz (2003), Taylor-Piliae and Froelicher (2004), and Yarcheski, Mahon, Yarcheski, and Cannella (2004).

Metaparadigm

Metaparadigm, broadly defined, is a term that sometimes is used when referring globally to the subject matter of greatest interest to members of a discipline. In nursing, the subject matter of greatest interest has been described and used in different ways by many writers. Therefore, although there appear to be consistent themes and patterns around which there is general agreement, there is not absolute consensus on whether or not nursing has, or needs to have, a metaparadigm. The issue is about boundaries that distinguish disciplines from one another, not so much in terms of subject matter (because certain subject matter may be of mutual interest to many disciplines) but in terms of how disciplines view and address the phenomena they see as central to their missions.

One direction in nursing has been to adopt a modification of what Yura and Torres (1975) introduced as the four most frequently recurring concepts (man, society, health, and nursing) in nursing theories and baccalaureate curricula as nursing's *metaparadigm concepts* (Fawcett, 1984). Fawcett (2000) describes nursing's *metaparadigm* (person, environment, health, and nursing) as "the most abstract component of the structural hierarchy of nursing knowledge" whose global concepts and propositions differentiate the discipline's domain from that of other disciplines, encompassing all phenomena of interest in a "perspective-neutral" way that is "international in scope and substance" (p. 4). In a logically deductive manner, the metaparadigm informs other elements of the hierarchy as the "schema for analysis of the content of conceptual models of nursing and nursing theories" (Fawcett, 2000, p. 6). Other nursing authors encourage independence from a priori ideas in theory development and more inductive case-by-case approaches to the evaluation of

M

conceptual models and theories in order to discover the meanings that each writer brings to the work.

The assumption is that concepts do not have universal meanings that are independent from the theoretical contexts in which they are used; and since their meanings will vary according to their use, agreement on the general importance of a set of predefined concepts is not the place to start. See, for example, H. S. Kim's (2000) work, which uses *metaparadigm* in a different way to refer to a boundary-setting typology of four conceptual domains (client, client-nurse, practice, and environment) that may support theory development. See also discussions of theory analysis and evaluation by Barnum (1998) and Meleis (1997), who do not use the notion of *metaparadigm* in their work. Barnum, however, associates efforts to identify general areas of agreement with attempts to define a universal theory of nursing; she contrasts this way of thinking with her notions about *commonplaces* (common topics addressed by most theories), which she says cannot be predetermined for every theory of nursing:

> Theory analysts create their own sets of commonplaces, and there is no one right set. . . . Because these terms [the metaparadigm concepts—*person, nursing, health, environment*] are commonplaces, and their definitions will vary from one theory to another, they cannot produce a universal theory (pp. 7, 9).

See **Theory.**

Metasynthesis

A *metasynthesis* is a qualitative critical appraisal of a body of literature in response to a particular question for the purpose of (a) providing an interpretation of conclusions based on the analysis and (b) adding a new perspective on the topic that builds upon the results of the review. This is a type of research study that requires the use of well-articulated and rigorously applied *metasummary* and *metasynthesis* techniques. *Metasummary* techniques (which constitute a type of *content analysis) involve strategies for extracting, editing, grouping, and abstracting findings, including calculation of frequency and intensity of effect sizes. Metasummary processes prepare quantitatively aggregated qualitative findings in a targeted domain for the interpretive integration of metasynthesis. *Metasynthesis* techniques involve a range of strategies, such as, taxonomic analysis, critical reflection, focused comparison, translation and synthesis of concepts, and use of imported concepts to integrate findings. A series of articles by Sandelowski and Barroso that examine motherhood in the context of maternal HIV infection, based on an integrative review and interpretive analysis of qualitative research report findings, provides detailed accounts of these processes (Sandelowski &

M

Barroso, 2002a, 2002b, 2003a, 2003b, 2003c; Sandlowski, Lambe, & Barroso, 2004).

The underlying purpose of the above-cited reports was to develop a "comprehensive, usable, and communicable protocol for conducting qualitative metasyntheses of health-related studies, [with] studies of women with HIV/AIDS [serving as] the method case" (Sandelowski & Barroso, 2002b, p. 2). In the process of conducting this methodological research, the authors created a typology to classify studies in accordance with the interpretive distance (level of abstraction) of the findings from the data (Sandelowski & Barroso, 2003a). This typology, and a similar typology for classifying qualitative research findings developed earlier by Kearney (2001b), provide a greater appreciation of the differing degrees of complexity found across all types of qualitative reports. The use of well-developed methods for metasythesis of qualitative studies has the potential to make combined results of qualitative research in particular areas more visible in the evidence-based practice literature/databases, where currently meta-analysis is used as the primary synthesizing method for clinical trial studies.

Metatheory

Metatheory is a theory about theory and is concerned with generating knowledge and debate within a discipline around broad issues, such as the nature of theory in general, the types of theory needed by the discipline, theory-building processes, suitable criteria for analyzing and evaluating theory, and guidelines for theory use in practice.

Many metatheoretical debates in nursing have focused on identifying the theory needs of a practice discipline (e.g., Carper, 1978; Dickoff, James, & Wiedenbach, 1968a, 1968b; Wald & Leonard, 1964; Wooldridge, Schmitt, Skipper, & Leonard, 1983). Later foci have included discussions about ontological and epistemological issues (Mitchell & Cody, 1992) and postmodernism (Reed, 1995; Watson, J., 1995) in nursing knowledge development. Barnum's (1998) work, *Nursing Theory: Analysis, Application, Evaluation* and Thorne and Hayes's (1997) edited volume on *Nursing Praxis* are further examples of metatheory. See also Fawcett's (2003a, 2003b) scholarly dialogues with Parker and with Cody (2003) on the topic of the relationship between theory and practice.

See Theory.

Method and Methodology

M

The terms *method* and *methodology* are often used in place of one another. For example, either term may be used as a section heading in a research report or as a chapter title in a dissertation. In that section or chapter the investigator describes in as much detail as space allows the design of the study and the actual procedures carried out in the collection and the analysis of the data. It would be useful, however, to distinguish between method (set of techniques or procedures used to collect and analyze data) and methodology (study of the theoretical and epistemological assumptions that guide the choice/use of a method). Particular methods (techniques and procedures) may be common to a number of research approaches that differ importantly from one another in methodology. Crotty (1998) makes such a distinction between methods (procedures and techniques) and methodology (action plan/design that determines method choice).

See **Research.**

Methodological Research

Methodological research is research on the tools of research. The focus of most methodological research is on the development of valid and reliable instruments that can later be used in substantive research. (A small amount of methodological research is concerned with issues of design and/or analysis.) There is a need in many kinds of nursing research to accurately measure cognitive and physical functioning or emotional responses of people. In some instances, instruments developed in other disciplines, for example, psychological profiles, life satisfaction or quality of life inventories, and the like, will serve the research purposes. In other instances, new or substantially revised instruments are created by investigators who want a scale, interview schedule, or observational method that will more specifically fit nursing practice.

For recent prototypical examples of methodological research in the nursing literature, see Cho (2003), H. C. W. Li and Lopez (2004), and Meretoja, Isoaho, and Leino-Kilpi (2004). See also Sandelowski and Barroso (2002b, 2003a, 2003c) for an example of a methodological research project involving creation of a protocol for conducting qualitative metasyntheses of health-related studies.

Middle-Range Theory

Middle-range, or *midrange theory,* deals with some part of a discipline's concerns related to particular topics, for example, pain management, rehabilitation, or death and dying. The scope is narrower than that of broad-range or grand theories; that is, it is at a greater level of concreteness and specificity (although not as narrow as *microtheory*). Liehr and M. J. Smith (1999) proposed a subclassification of high-middle, middle, and low-middle based on a theory's scope and level of abstraction. However, at either end of this continuum the appropriateness of identifying a theory as middle-range (versus grand or micro-range) may be debated (McEwen & Wills, 2002).

M

Fawcett (2000) has identified Orlando's theory of deliberative nursing process, Peplau's theory of interpersonal relations, and Watson's theory of human caring as examples of middle-range nursing theories. Liehr and M. J. Smith (1999) identified 22 more-recent theories as "the middle range theory foundation" and added to these in a later collection of selected works (Smith, M. J., & Liehr, 2003). Some of these include Mishel's theory of uncertainty in illness, Reed's theory of self-transcendence, Jezewski's theory of culture brokering, Good and Moore's pain management theory (balance between analgesia and side effects), Resnick's theory of self-efficacy, and LoBiondo-Wood's theory of family stress and adaptation.

See **Theory.**

Missing Data

The problem of *missing data* plagues almost all of quantitative nursing research. It is the rare experiment, correlational study, or survey that has complete data for every subject for every variable. Some subjects drop out of a study before it is completed. Some omit certain items on questionnaires. Some instruments break down. Some records are lost. Some clerks fail to enter the appropriate data for various participants. And so on.

What to do about it? There is a vast literature concerned with suggestions ranging all the way from "forget about it" to fancy statistical procedures for estimating what the missing data "might have been."

The best approach, of course, is to try to minimize the occurrence of any missing data by, for example, urging every participant to provide a response to every question on a survey. The next best is to use some sort of 'imputation' strategy, in which one or more estimates are calculated for the missing data. The third best strategy is to use some sort of 'deletion' strategy (resulting in even more missing data!). The worst strategy is to ignore the problem by not even providing in the research report any indication of how the missing data problem was handled.

For descriptions of various methods for handling missing data, see Little and Rubin (2002) and Allison (2001). And for a good example of the reporting of how missing data were handled in a substantive study, see Murphy, Chung, and Johnson (2002).

See **Deletion** and **Imputation.**

Mixed Methods Research

Mixed methods research is a term associated with research that uses a combination of methods usually identified with qualitative research and methods that are usually identified with quantitative research (see, for example, Creswell, 2003) It should not be confused with the terms *mixed models* or *mixed effects* that are used in other contexts such as the analysis of variance.

M

It is important to understand that the use of a mixed methods approach does not make research better or more *valid than the use of either a qualitative or a quantitative approach. Choice of a research design always is dependent on the research question. It also should be understood that some mixed methods designs are by nature predominantly qualitative or predominantly quantitative. Creswell (2003) describes six mixed methods strategies and identifies criteria for selecting among them as follows.

> (1) What is the implementation sequence of the quantitative and qualitative data collection in the proposed study? (2) What priority will be given to the quantitative and qualitative data collection and analysis? (3) At what stage in the research project will the quantitative and qualitative data and findings be integrated? (4) Will an overall theoretical perspective (e.g., gender, race/ethnicity, lifestyle, class) be used in the study? (p. 211).

For a nursing research example of the use of conceptual triangulation in a mixed methods research framework, see Dabbs et al. (2004).
See **Triangulation.**

Mode

The *mode* of a set of data for a variable is that value of the variable that occurs more often than any other value in the data.

Model

A *model* is a graphic or symbolic representation of a phenomenon that serves to objectify and present a certain perspective or point of view about its nature and/or function. Various media are employed in the construction of models, ranging from three-dimensional objects (such as plastic models of human organs and chemical structures found in the biological and physical sciences) to diagrams, geometric forms, mathematical formulas/equations, and words.

Physical models mirror a phenomenon in form and structure, but on a smaller scale. A path diagram is an example of a *semantic model,* that is, a reduction of a hypothesis to statistical symbols (a causal model) for purposes of analysis. Similarly, *conceptual models* are statements, or groups of statements, that attempt to model a view of the nature and interrelated aspects of a phenomenon. There are many conceptual models of nursing.

These models may be *pre-theoretic* (representing preliminary theorizing that provides a descriptive and philosophical base for later more formal theorizing) or *post-theoretic* (used within a theory to illustrate the structure of relationships or major features of the theory). Some authors

M

encourage a distinction between pre-theoretic *conceptual models* and post-theoretic *theoretic models*. Other authors consider conceptual models and theoretic models to be similar structurally, being composed of interrelated concepts that make up a whole, with theoretic models connoting 'less tentativeness' than conceptual models (Chinn & Kramer, 1995, p. 219). Additionally, the terms *theoretical model/framework* and *theory* are often used interchangeably. Again, some authors distinguish between models, in the schematic sense, which precede and coexist with theory, and theories, which provide fuller explanations of the phenomena in question.

Moderator Variable

A *moderator variable* is a variable that alters the relationship between two other variables. It is therefore indicative of an interaction effect.

The term is often used synonymously with *mediating variable* but should not be. As indicated in the entry for *mediating variable,* Baron and Kenny (1986), Lindley and Walker (1993), and J. A. Bennett (2000) all provide excellent discussions of the difference between moderators and mediators.

Example: Sex might very well act as a moderator variable for the relationship between height and weight. For adult males the correlation between height and weight might be high and positive, whereas for adult females the correlation between height and weight might also be positive, but low.

Modernism

Modernism (the modern *worldview) is a response to *modernity* (a cultural movement that began in the renaissance with the rise of secularization, industrialism, and the scientific revolution). It is a broad term for an overall intellectual, social, cultural, scientific, and artistic climate throughout today's Westernized world. Modernism is most easily defined narrowly in relation to specific events or movements, such as trends in 'modern' lifestyles, science, philosophy, literature, music, architecture, and all the art forms as well as reactions to political, environmental, or economic events and happenings. Attempts to define it more broadly elicit a wide range of opinions, such as those that characterize the 'modern' age as one of scientific discovery, the rise of consumerism, breaks with tradition, experimentation, and movement toward streamlining and simplification in terms of both the material culture and lifestyle. There also are opposing schools among the many modernist traditions in art, literary criticism, and philosophy, referred to as *classical modernism* and *neomodernism* (variously described as a new movement, a reaction

M

against the dominance of modernism, and a suspicion of postmodernism). However, most often, *modernism* and *neomodernism* are defined in relation to *postmodernism.*

See **Postmodernism.**

Multicollinearity

Multicollinearity (some authors drop the 'multi') is a problem sometimes encountered in multiple regression analysis when the independent variables are very highly correlated with one another. In the extreme case, one of the independent variables may itself be a linear composite of two or more of the other independent variables, and this will make it impossible to actually carry out the analysis (the matrix of intercorrelations among the independent variables is said to be 'singular').

Example: If Score on Part 1, Score on Part 2, and Total Score were all included as independent variables in a regression analysis there would be a multicollinearity problem, because Total Score is equal to Score on Part 1 plus Score on Part 2 and therefore provides redundant information.

Multivariate Analysis

The term *multivariate analysis* usually applies to any statistical procedure that involves more than two variables. However, some authors insist that the term is appropriate only for analysis of multiple *dependent* variables, and they would not refer to multiple regression analysis (one dependent variable, any number of independent variables) or factor analysis (in which the independent vs. dependent distinction is not relevant) as multivariate.

To make matters even more confusing, hardly anyone calls 'one-way' analysis of variance a multivariate procedure, as there is just one independent variable (often a 'treatment' variable having several categories or 'levels') and one dependent variable (some sort of 'response' or 'criterion' variable in which the researcher is primarily interested). However, if the independent variable has three or more categories, if these categories are 'coded' into two or more 'dummy' variables, and if multiple regression analysis (which is mathematically equivalent to the analysis of variance) is employed in the analysis of the data, there *are* more than two variables and the people who take the less restrictive view of the term should regard the analysis as multivariate.

The most common multivariate analyses are multivariate analysis of variance (one or more nominal independent variables and two or more interval dependent variables), discriminant analysis (just the opposite, i.e., two or more interval independent variables and one or more nominal dependent variables), and canonical correlation analysis (two or

M

more independent variables and two or more dependent variables, all of which are usually of interval level). See McLaughlin and Marascuilo (1990) or any multivariate text for details.

Multivariate analysis is currently a fashionable buzz word. Researchers are thought to be really "with it" if they use some sort of multivariate analysis, because many variables impinge on a given problem. However, it always has been, and always will be, "researcher's choice" regarding the number of variables she or he wants to study, just as long as they are relevant to the research questions. If a particular scientist chooses to study *only* obesity, say, or *only* the effect of the reduction of cigarette smoking *on* obesity, that scientist should feel free to do so and should resist pressures to include any additional variables.

Example: A defensible analysis of the research question "What is the effect of amount of salary increase on nurses' satisfaction and performance?" should consider satisfaction and performance in the *same* analysis, as they may be correlated with one another. It would be inappropriate to undertake two analyses, one with salary increase as independent and satisfaction as dependent, and the other with salary increase as independent and performance as dependent.

M

N

Narrative Inquiry

Narrative inquiry is the analysis of meaning in context through interpretation of persons' life experiences in the form of storytelling for the purpose of evoking a response from readers and promoting dialogue. Frank (2004) describes it as a type of truth telling where 'truth' is seen as offering solely partial perspectives.

> [T]he postmodern sense of truth does not require an explanation that counts as a solution; postmodern truth sees too many perspectives to accept the closure of explanation. . . . [But the narrative conveys the] power to see what is and to *say* what is [in ways that help us to overcome] our innate fear of complexity . . . [by] realizing what truth needs to be told (pp. 439–440).

Nursing examples of narrative inquiry are Bailey's (2004) analysis of chronic obstructive pulmonary disease (COPD) patients' stories of breathlessness ("It's scary/When you can't breathe") and Dombeck's (2003) examination of how nurses understand their professional culture and their professional personhood "in the context of the images of nursing in the society at large" (p. 351).

Narrow-Range Theory

Chinn and Kramer (1995) describe *narrow-range theories,* or *micro-theories,* as those that deal with a limited range of discrete phenomena that are specifically defined and are not expanded to include their link with the broad concerns of a discipline (p. 122). Higgins and Moore (2000) propose two levels of micro-range theory.

> At the higher level, micro-range theory is closely related to [*]middle-range theory but is comprised of 1 or 2 major [*]concepts, and its application frequently is limited to a particular event; for example, theories related to

decubitus or catheter care. At the lower level, micro-range theory is defined as a set of working hypotheses or propositions . . . [that are not part
of] a formal theoretical system (p. 181).

Some authors equate narrow-range micro-theory with *practice theory,*
but others "maintain that all nursing theory, regardless of level, is practice theory" (Higgins & Moore, p. 182).
See Theory.

Naturalistic Inquiry

Naturalistic inquiry refers to the study of phenomena in their natural settings, as in *fieldwork/field research. It is a general characteristic of
many types of qualitative research. The underlying idea is that the researcher goes to learn about study participants in their natural environments rather than bringing them into the researcher's environment.
"Historically, analysts have distinguished between experimental (laboratory) and field (natural) research settings, hence the argument that qualitative research is naturalistic" (Denzin & Lincoln, 2000, p. 24).

Needs Assessment/Need Analysis

Needs assessment or *need analysis* uses a problem-solving process for the
purpose of collecting, organizing, and presenting information that describes the needs of a target population and evaluates their importance
relative to demand. A variety of methods may be used, including inventories, surveys, statistical measures, cost analysis, utilization analysis,
and interviews with groups and key informants. Needs assessments are
undertaken by agencies and service organizations for a variety of reasons: in connection with decisions to expand services, write proposals to
obtain program funding, adapt to changing needs of consumers, attract
additional types of clients, set budget priorities, or implement new procedures. For example, see Davidson, Cockburn, Daly, and Fisher's
(2004) discussion of a rationale for development of a needs assessment
instrument for patients with heart failure and Bashore's (2004) report of
a needs assessment to determine what childhood and adolescent cancer
survivors in a Life After Cancer Program knew about their disease and
effects of treatment. See also Soriano (1995) and Altschuld and Witkin
(1999) for further information about conducting needs assessments and
developing solution strategies.
See Evaluation Research and Problem Solving.

Negative Case Analysis

In qualitative research, a *negative case* is an exception or variation—a
case that does not fit into existing categories or support relationship
statements (i.e., hypotheses). Actively searching for and analyzing negative

cases is important. They produce variation in the data that deepens understanding by disconfirming or broadening previously held ideas and generating new insights. They also increase the *validity of findings and strengthen theory development by identifying needs to reexamine and revise the analysis and suggesting new directions to pursue in data collection. Olshansky (1996) discusses the usefulness of negative cases in her clinical practice and research on infertility. She notes:

> Over time . . . I also began to see that conflicting findings contributed to a more detailed and comprehensive understanding of the phenomenon under study, and, as researchers we would do well to embrace such seemingly conflicting findings in an effort to reflect the multiple realities of the persons we are trying to understand (p. 402).

Negative Relationship

A *negative relationship* between two variables, say X and Y, is one in which Y increases as X decreases and Y decreases as X increases. It is also called an inverse relationship.

If the Pearson product-moment correlation coefficient is used to measure the relationship between two variables, a negative relationship is indicated by a number between −1 and 0.

A common confusion is to think of a negative relationship as *no* relationship (because of the word 'negative'). A negative relationship of −.70 is actually a stronger relationship than a positive relationship of +.50.

Example: There is a negative relationship between bowling scores and golf scores; that is, as golf scores go down bowling scores tend to go up. Note, however, that this is simply an artifact of how the two games are scored. The two *traits,* bowling ability and golf ability, are actually positively related. The reader is cautioned to be on the lookout for that same sort of phenomenon when interpreting negative correlation coefficients that are reported in nursing research.

Neomodernism
See **Modernism.**

Nominal Scale

A *nominal scale* is a level of scientific measurement consisting of a set of unordered categories. Any numbers can be used as labels for the categories.

Examples: Religious affiliation is a typical nominal scale. Each person being 'measured' for religious affiliation is given a number that is a label for a category (e.g., Protestant = 2), but the numbers have no other numerical interpretation, such as one religion being better than another.

See **Scale.**

Nomothetic

Nomothetic analysis is concerned with finding general laws that sub-sume individual cases. It involves generalizing from one case to a larger group of which it is thought to be representative, or comparing the single case with another group in order to identify the differences. *Nomothetic generalizations* state the results of such analyses.

See **Case Study** and **Generalizations.**

Nonparametric Statistics

Nonparametric statistics are inferential statistical procedures that do not make any assumptions about the shape of the population distribution and do not place any restrictions on its parameters.

They are to be contrasted with parametric statistics, such as the 'pooled' *t* test of the significance of the difference between means of two independent samples, which assumes that the corresponding populations have normal distributions and equal variances. There are two common misconceptions regarding nonparametric statistics. The first is that they are used for small samples. The second is that they are descriptive statistics rather than inferential statistics. These confusions may result from the understanding that for small samples it is inappropriate to use the sample variances and the normal sampling distribution to test differences between means (the sample variances might provide poor estimates of the population variances), and because of the close association between certain descriptive statistics, such as Spearman's rank correlation coefficient or Kendall's tau, with nonparametric inference.

One of the principal sourcebooks for nonparametric techniques is Siegel and Castellan (1988).

Example: One of the most popular nonparametric statistics is the Mann-Whitney *U* Test for two independent samples, in which the differences between ranks are examined rather than the differences between actual scores (see Landis et al., 2003, for an example of its use).

Nonrecursive Model

In path analysis and structural equation modeling a *nonrecursive model* is one in which some of the causal relationships are postulated to be reciprocal.

See **Path Analysis** and **Structural Equation Modeling.**

Null Hypothesis

A *null hypothesis* is a specific conjecture regarding the value of a population parameter that is usually postulated for the express purpose of being rejected by the sample data.

There are two reasons for the modifier 'null': (a) the hope that the hypothesis gets 'nullified' by the data and (b) the fact that most null hypotheses claim that some parameter is equal to zero.

Example: There is no relationship between age and pulse rate.

Number Needed To Treat/To Harm

After the results of a clinical trial have been reported, the *number needed to treat* (NNT) can be calculated as the reciprocal of the attributable risk (see entry for *risk*) and is interpreted as the number of subjects that would have to be exposed to the 'treatment' in order to produce one additional occurrence of the event (outcome) that serves as the dependent variable. The term 'number needed to treat' is usually replaced by the term 'number needed to harm' (NNH) if the event is a negative event such as death.

O

Objective/Objectivity

In the history of scientific inquiry, the term *objective* has represented the ideal of observations and judgments that are free and independent from personal reflections, opinions, and feelings. Thus, *objectivity* has become known as the valued polar opposite of *subjectivity*. However, there is not agreement that such objectivity, especially in the social/human sciences, is possible or even desirable. Observations are felt by many to be *theory-laden* in the sense that they do not exist independent from the theoretical contexts that define them. Over time, there also has been increasing recognition of the role of subjectivity (researchers' judgments based on training and experience) in shaping the meaning, values, and discourses that guide research projects from initial design to final outcome. Consequently, while researchers may entertain different notions about the meaning of *objectivity* as it pertains to their work, there continues to be movement away from thinking in terms of dichotomies *(objectivity versus subjectivity)* to thinking about relationships between *objectivity and subjectivity* in approaches to scientific inquiry.

See **Subjective/Subjectivity** and **Objectivism**.

Objectivism

Objectivism is the epistemological view that there have to be certain basic sorts of knowledge that will always be true regardless of individuals' thoughts or desires. That is, there is a known world "out there" (object) that is independent of the knower (subject). Therefore, the investigator (subject) can study the object without influencing it or being influenced by it and discover the objective truth as long as procedures to control for bias are rigorously upheld. Objectivism is the underpinning of *positivism/postpositivism.

See **Epistemology**, **Subjectivism**, and **Constructivism/Constructionalism**.

Observation

The term *observation* is used in two different senses in nursing theory and research. One meaning refers to a procedure for gathering data that requires the investigator to witness and record certain behaviors. The other meaning refers to a piece of data, as in "The total number of observations for this study was 73."

In the former sense of the term, the modifiers 'participant' and 'nonparticipant' are sometimes used to indicate the level of involvement of the investigator in the study environment.

In the latter sense, an observation may be 'univariate' or 'multivariate'; that is, it may be a measurement taken on a single variable or a set of measurements taken on several variables. In any statistical analysis it is essential that the observations be independent—that there is a one-to-one correspondence between subject and observation. It is very common for researchers to collect data in such a way that some subjects are counted in the data once, others are counted twice, still others are counted five or more times, and so forth. That creates havoc with many tests of statistical significance, such as the chi-square test, for which one of the assumptions is the independence of the observations.

Example: Obstetric nurses interested in the behavior of mothers when feeding their newborn babies might unobtrusively observe such behavior and record the number of smiles or hugs, whether or not or for how long a time the mother 'coos' to the child, and so forth. The resulting data then become the observations that can be subjected to one or more statistical analyses. Thus in the same study the word 'observation' could be used in both of its senses.

Odds Ratio

An *odds ratio* is a summary index usually associated with the results of a case-control study, and is calculated by dividing the odds of exposure for the 'cases' who contract the 'disease' that is of concern by the odds of exposure for the 'controls' who did not contract the disease (or occasionally the other way 'round, i.e., the odds for the controls divided by the odds for the cases). It is a good approximation to the relative risk for rare diseases.

One-Tailed Test

A *one-tailed test* is a test of statistical significance in which the null hypothesis is pitted against a directional alternative hypothesis. A one-tailed test would be used if the alternative hypothesis to a null hypothesis of no relationship were a hypothesis of a positive relationship.

See **Alternative Hypothesis, Null Hypothesis,** and **Test of Significance.**

Ontology

The term *ontology* refers to the study/philosophy of being (i.e., its nature or kinds of existence). In conjunction with *epistemology* (views on how we know what we know), it informs theoretical perspectives and methodologies that guide scientific research. ". . . [That is], each theoretical perspective [underlying a particular research methodology] embodies a certain way of understanding *what is* (ontology) as well as a certain way of understanding *what it means to know* (epistemology)" (Crotty, 1998, p. 10).

See **Realism, Idealism,** and **Relativism.**

Operational Definition

An *operational definition* links theoretical constructs with the real world by identifying what phenomena (empirical indicators/referents) will be observed and how they will be measured. Concrete ideas (e.g., weight, blood pressure, touch, activities of daily living, fluid intake) are not too difficult to operationalize because empirical indicators can be specified with some precision and direct measurements may be made. However, research concerns in nursing frequently involve abstract notions (e.g., social support, self-esteem, adaptation, sensory deprivation, body image, health, or well-being) that do not have exact empirical indicators and can only be measured indirectly. Complex and abstract concepts have many aspects. Operationalization thus becomes a process of sorting out aspects and choosing which one(s) to feature in the research. For example, Long, Ritter, and Gonzalez (2003) operationalized "disease self-management" by an experimental treatment called Tomando in their community-based study of the health of Hispanics.

The investigator is free to choose one method or multiple methods of measurement. Even so, the process of operationalization in a single piece of research will often limit to some extent the number of ways in which variables may be explored. The least limiting approaches to operationalization involve qualitative methods aimed at producing rich description. Such methods involve a very broad range of observation and measurement styles. Thus, they often do not involve narrow operational definitions that would preclude description of the different ways in which the variables of interest manifest themselves. Other types of research require a more restricted focus, which means that the researcher must choose to feature some aspects and ignore or downplay others.

It is not unusual for other people to question or disagree with the way in which investigators have operationalized constructs. Nevertheless, a benefit of a precise operational definition lies in its ability to clearly communicate the researcher's perception of, for example, anxiety, within the context of the particular research. The implications of research results are also clearer when examined in the light of this established framework. No delimited set of operational definitions or single piece of research can account for the complexity of some constructs. Careful operationalization of constructs, however, can help to provide meaningful insights on which further research may build.

O

Oral History

Oral history captures original thoughts and meanings that are woven into spoken accounts of personal experiences. Historians and biographers collect oral histories in order to preserve valuable primary data that also enable them to place information from stories about the phenomenon of interest in historical and cultural context. "The primary purpose of oral history is historical preservation . . . [but oral history techniques also may provide] a means of advocacy for the populations that nurses serve" (Taft et al., 2004, p. 39). See, for example, Fairman and Mahon's (2001) oral history of Florence Downs, a well-recognized nursing leader; Madsen's (2003) report of an oral history project examining possible factors contributing to the phasing out of private duty nursing in Australia; and Taft et al.'s (2004) oral history intervention with elders in nursing home and community settings involving the recording of their memories of World War II.

See **Biographical Method** and **Historical Research.**

Ordinal Scale

An *ordinal scale* is a level of scientific measurement consisting of a set of ordered categories. The numbers used as labels for the categories signify relative order but not quantity. The numbers can be transformed into any other numbers that are in the same order as the original numbers (e.g., 2, 3, 4, 5, 7 are just as appropriate as 1, 2, 3, 4, 5).

Example: A typical ordinal scale is a Likert scale with the categories strongly agree, agree, undecided, disagree, and strongly disagree.

See **Likert Scale** and **Scale.**

Orthogonal Design/Rotation/Contrasts

The term *orthogonal* is used in at least three different senses in research, all of which have the general connotation of *independent* or *unrelated.*

An orthogonal design is a balanced design in which all main effects and all interaction effects can be assessed independently of one another.

An orthogonal rotation in factor analysis is a transformation of factor loadings in such a way that the underlying factors remain uncorrelated with one another.

Orthogonal contrasts are comparisons carried out in the analysis of variance such that the result of one comparison has no influence on the result of another comparison. For example, a contrast of Christians versus Jews and a contrast of Catholics versus Protestants are orthogonal because the second contrast involves the comparisons of two religions on "opposite sides of the ledger" that were on the "same side of the ledger" in the first contrast.

Outcomes Research

Outcomes research, according to the Agency for Healthcare Research and Quality (AHRQ), "evaluates the impact of health care on health outcomes of patients and populations" (Stryer, Siegel, & Rodgers, 2004, p. III-1). It often uses large data sets on real-world populations, thus enhancing the representativeness and generalizability of findings. An example is Aiken, Clarke, Cheung, Sloane, and Silber (2003) analysis of outcomes data for 232,342 hospital patients discharged from all of the nonfederal hospitals in a large U.S. state, linked to administrative and survey data providing information on educational composition, staffing, and other characteristics. An important finding was that surgical patients in hospitals with higher proportions of nurses educated at the baccalaureate level or higher experienced lower mortality and failure-to-rescue rates. Data collection was then expanded internationally to England, Scotland, Germany, and three Canadian provinces (Clarke, 2004). The term *outcomes research* has more recently been applied in the context of outcomes management in health care organizations. Ingersoll (2005) defines outcomes research as "the use of rigorous scientific methods to measure the effect of some intervention on some outcome or outcomes (Ingersoll, 1998) . . . [in order to] . . . establish care delivery standards and to develop policy statements about best practices" (p. 307). See also Polit and Beck's (2004) discussion of outcomes research.

See **Health Services Research.**

Outlier

An *outlier* is a data point that appears to be isolated from the other data points and may therefore be the result of an unusual measurement error.

It is very common in scientific research to employ some sort of procedure to try to identify outliers and to retain them, correct them (if they are wrong), or delete them from the data analysis. The reason is that even a single outlier can have a profound effect on the determination of a mean, a standard deviation, a correlation coefficient, or any of a number of statistics that may be used to summarize the research findings, particularly if the sample size is small.

Example: If measurements of the number of children in ten families yield the values 0, 0, 1, 2, 2, 2, 3, 3, 5, and 22, the 22 should be carefully checked to see if a reporting or recording error might have been made (perhaps it should have been 2 but that digit was inadvertently repeated). Otherwise the results could be quite distorted. With the outlier the mean would be 4; without it the mean would be 2. The differences in the standard deviations in the two cases would be even more pronounced, and if that variable were to be correlated with a variable for which the 22 were paired with another outlying value, that single data point could 'anchor' the correlation coefficient at an artificially high level.

P

Paradigm

The *paradigm* concept was introduced by the philosopher Thomas Kuhn (1922–1996) in his work on the nature of scientific change. It refers to patterns or systems of beliefs *(worldviews)* about science and knowledge production occurring within and across disciplines. For Kuhn, a discipline's paradigm (or *disciplinary matrix*) dictates what views of reality (ontology), knowledge forms/theory (epistemology), and processes of scientific investigation (methodology) are acceptable. That is, it will contain:

1. Concepts, theories, assumptions, beliefs, values, and principles that form a way for the discipline to interpret the subject matter with which it is concerned.

2. Research methods considered to be best suited to generating knowledge within this frame of reference.

3. What is open to investigation—priorities and views on knowledge-deficit areas where research and theory-building is most needed.

4. What is closed to inquiry for a time.

By this definition, it is similar to an action plan that describes the work to be done in a discipline and how it will be accomplished. Evolutionism, structuralism, functionalism, economic determinism, and psychoanalytic theory are examples of paradigms that, at various times, have been influential in shaping the agendas of scientific disciplines. For Kuhn, science in a discipline develops through revolutionary processes of *convergence* around an agreed-upon paradigm and periods of *crisis* resulting in the replacement of the dominant paradigm by another. A discipline whose worldview of itself and its approach to its subject matter changes from one understanding to a radically different one is said to have undergone a *paradigm shift* (as experienced by physics around the time of Einstein).

Kuhn's views about the characteristics and powerfulness of paradigms have generated much debate among adherents and critics; and the many usages of *paradigm* (including Kuhn's various treatments of the concept) have resulted in some vagueness and an aura of ambiguity around this term. Most generally, *paradigm talk* refers to dialogues surrounding different schools of thought, each of which may be described in terms of its *knowledge claims* (i.e., ontology, epistemology, theoretical perspective, and methodology). Lincoln and Guba (2000) and Creswell (2003) provide good discussions of the knowledge claims of some of these *inquiry paradigms* (positivism, postpositivism, critical theory, constructivism, advocacy/participatory, and pragmatism).

A number of practice and social science fields are thought of as *multiparadigm disciplines* because there are a variety of different ways to understand their domains and the phenomena that are central to their intellectual and social missions. Nursing, for instance, has been influenced by paradigms from many other fields, such as stress and adaptation, psychoanalytic, systems, developmental, organizational, and role theories; symbolic interaction; and holism (Meleis, 1997).

The presence of *competing paradigms* within and across disciplines can spur progress and encourage enlightened dialogue; but perceived hegemony (dominance of one paradigm over others) produces controversy. The latter figures in what were once fashionable to refer to as *the paradigm debates* surrounding 'qualitative' and 'quantitative' approaches. Discussion focused on the *incommensurability* of these two 'paradigms,' which, because they operate within different worldviews, makes direct comparisons to determine which is 'best' impossible. To overlook the many paradigmatic allegiances of approaches identified as 'quantitative' or 'qualitative' in order to create a dichotomy (two opposing paradigms) could be seen as an oversimplification. However, this type of debate signals a response from those who would champion an ideal of greater tolerance of methodological diversity and support for *paradigmatic pluralism* (an attitude of acceptance within and across disciplines of different paradigms that may be used to direct scientific work in an atmosphere where no paradigm dominates the others).

See **Worldview.**

Parallel Forms

The *parallel forms* technique is a method for assessing the reliability of a measuring instrument that has two or more interchangeable operationalizations, e.g., two forms of a spelling test, where each form consists of 50 words drawn at random from an unabridged dictionary.

See **Reliability.**

Parameter

In statistics, the term *parameter* has one and only one meaning, and that is a descriptive index of a population (a population mean, population standard deviation, population correlation coefficient, etc.). Population parameters are constants that are usually unknown but are hypothesized about or estimated from sample data.

The term causes a great deal of difficulty because in mathematics a parameter is not a constant but a variable (*x* is a function of *t*, *y* is a function of *t*, and the like), and some researchers use the term in a similar sense to refer to a dimension that is of direct concern in the problem that is being investigated (e.g., "The parameters we are interested in are sex, age, height, and weight").

In more general parlance a parameter is some sort of boundary condition ("Within what parameters are we permitted to operate?"). That meaning derives primarily from confusion with the word *perimeter,* however.

Another context in which the term *parameter* arises is in computer programming. In that context a parameter is a piece of information that needs to be specified for the software to execute a command.

It is the statistical meaning that is most commonly encountered in nursing research.

Example: An interesting, but unknown, parameter is the percentage of American nurses who smoke cigarettes. It has been estimated in a number of studies (see, e.g., Wagner, 1985) but no one really knows how small or how large that percentage actually is.

Partial Correlation Coefficient

A *partial correlation coefficient* is a special type of correlation coefficient that indicates the magnitude and direction of the relationship between two variables with one or more other variables statistically controlled ('partialed out'). It is to be contrasted with a zero-order correlation coefficient, which does not involve any 'partialing.' If one variable has been statistically controlled, the coefficient is called a first-order partial coefficient; if two variables have been statistically controlled, the coefficient is called a second-order partial coefficient, and so forth.

There is also such a thing as a semipartial correlation coefficient, which, as the name implies, involves statistical control with respect to one of the two variables but not the other.

Partial correlations were used by Walker and Montgomery (1994) in their study of maternal identity and role attainment.

See Zero-Order Correlation Coefficient.

Participant Observation

Participant observation is the central technique used in ethnographic fieldwork. It involves direct observation of everyday life in study participants' natural settings and participation in their 'lifeways' and activities as much as possible. Extensive fieldnotes are maintained that account for the words and actions of all involved, including the researcher; the context of recorded situations; and researcher thoughts and comments. Measures of adequacy are accuracy and completeness, sensitivity to use of language and nonverbal communication, attention to descriptive detail, and researcher self-awareness.

The degree to which a participant observer <u>engages</u> in activities versus <u>observes</u> activities, persons, and the physical aspects in the situation varies from study to study and over the course of a single study; but there should be an accounting. Although participant observation is part of fieldwork, its role often is assumed and under-reported in the literature. The following research reports comment on participant-observation activities: Cannaerts, de Casterlé, and Grypdonck (2004); Dombeck (2003); M. C. McCarthy (2003a, 2003b); Mohr (2004); Mueller (2004); B. A. Powers (2001); Tzeng and Lipson (2004).

See **Fieldnotes** and **Fieldwork.**

Participatory Action Research (PAR)

Participatory action research (PAR) is a broad term for several forms of *action research* identified by Kemmis and McTaggart (2000) as (a) *participatory research (PR)*—associated with "neo-Marxist approaches to community development . . . in the Third World", (b) *critical action research*—"represented in the literatures of educational action research . . . [and] committed to social analyses in the critical social science tradition that reveal . . . disempowerment and injustice," and (c) *classroom action research*—researcher-assisted individual judgments of teachers about how to improve their own practices based on "interpretive modes of inquiry and data collection" (pp. 568–569). It is a problem-solving approach entered into collaboratively by researchers and *stakeholders. Because it is not a unitary approach, however, PAR may involve different research processes and orientations to situations where the common theme is that participants

> want to make changes thoughtfully—that is, after critical reflection. It emerges when people want to think 'realistically' about where they are now, how things came to be that way, and, from these starting points, how, in practice, things might be changed (Kemmis & McTaggart, p. 573).

For nursing research examples see N. L. Anderson et al. (2001), Chalmers et al. (2004), and Crist (2002).

See **Action Research.**

Path Analysis

Path analysis is a special application of regression analysis. Prior to the actual carrying out of the regression analysis the researcher displays in a pictorial model (called a path diagram) the kinds of causal relationships that are alleged to hold. The regression analysis then provides some evidence regarding the plausibility of the model. It does not demonstrate that such causal relationships actually exist; it strengthens or weakens the *case* for causality.

The associated vocabulary for path analysis differs somewhat from the vocabulary of traditional regression analysis. Instead of independent and dependent variables one speaks of exogenous and endogenous variables. The former are those variables whose causes are not under investigation; the latter are those whose direct and indirect causes are of concern within the model. The magnitudes of the effects of the exogenous variables upon the endogenous variables, and of some of the endogenous variables upon other endogenous variables, are called path coefficients (they are actually partial regression coefficients—standardized or unstandardized). Models that postulate only one-way causation are called recursive; those that allow for reciprocal causation are called nonrecursive.

There are additional technical terms for specific aspects of path analysis, such as the matters of 'identification' and 'specification' (see Pedhazur, 1997, for details).

Example: A path analysis might be carried out to determine the direct effect of stress on depression as mediated by social support. Such a model is an integral part of many theories regarding the relationships among those variables (e.g., Norbeck, 1981) and can be diagrammed as follows:

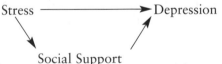

For more complicated, but more realistic, examples of path analyses in nursing research, see Smyth and Yarandi (1992) and Lucas, Atwood, and Hagaman (1993).

Patterns of Knowing

Carper's (1978) study of nursing literature revealed four fundamental *patterns of knowing,* i.e., shared, interrelated understandings that, as an integrated whole, constitute the knowledge base of the discipline. Chinn and Kramer (2004) have expanded Carper's descriptions of (a) empirical knowing, (b) ethical knowing, (c) personal knowing, and (d) aesthetic knowing by formally describing each pattern (conceptually or theoretically), addressing ways in which the patterns are expressed in practice, and proposing methods for developing each pattern. Thus, the *empiric pattern of knowing* involves developing and validating formal expressions of knowledge (theories and models) through programs of theory development and research to develop scientific competence. Development of the *ethical pattern of knowing* involves valuing and clarifying ethical situations to create formal expressions of ethical knowledge (principles and codes) that provide a foundation for moral/ethical comportment. Development of the *personal pattern of knowing* involves responsively and reflectively opening (consciously comprehending experiences and seeing oneself in them) and centering (focusing on inner feelings and perceptions of experiences) to create nondiscursive (genuine self) and discursive (autobiography/stories) forms of expression that demonstrate therapeutic use of self. The development of the *aesthetic pattern of knowing* involves processes of envisioning, rehearsing, and creating works of art that symbolize perceived meanings of nursing practice experiences and aesthetic criticism (reflective interpretation of art forms) that produce the collective affirmation from members of the discipline (appreciation and inspiration) that becomes reflected in transformative art/acts (integration of aesthetic, empiric, ethical, and personal patterns of knowing). Integration is important from a disciplinary perspective in that "[o]ne pattern of knowing by itself will not uncover all the knowledge needed for a human and practice-oriented science" (Meleis, 1997, p. 148). Also, Chinn and Kramer suggest that knowledge development or critical analysis of individual nursing situations that fail to integrate all the patterns of knowing "leads to uncritical acceptance, narrow interpretation, and partial utilization of knowledge. [They] call this *patterns gone wild* [because] when . . . the patterns are used in isolation from one another . . . the potential for synthesis of the whole is lost" (p. 13).

See **Empirical Knowing, Ethical Knowing, Personal Knowing,** and **Aesthetic Knowing.**

Pearson Product-Moment Correlation Coefficient ("Pearson *r*")

The *Pearson product-moment correlation coefficient,* affectionately known as Pearson *r,* is a statistic invented by the British statistician Karl Pearson for summarizing the magnitude and the direction of the linear relationship between two variables. It can take on any value between −1 (perfect inverse relationship) and +1 (perfect direct relationship).

Peer Debriefing

In qualitative research, *peer debriefing* involves seeking input (substantive or methodological) from knowledgeable colleagues as consultants, soliciting their reactions as listeners, and using them as sounding boards for the researcher's ideas. The researcher decides when and if peer debriefing will be helpful. Peer debriefing is not the same as quantitative researchers' use of multiple raters and expert panels. Individuals external to the research are not positioned to 'validate' interpretations that have been arrived at through close contact with and in-depth understanding of the data (Sandelowski, 1998).

Percentage

As is well known, a *percentage* is a number that indicates a part of the whole. It can take on any value between 0 (none) and 100 (all). Percentages over 100 are occasionally encountered in statements such as "The average salary for beginning staff nurses has increased by over 200% in the last three decades," but references to percentages greater than 100 are rarely found in nursing research reports.

Personal Knowing

The fundamental pattern of *personal knowing* involves a reflective, perceptive awareness of self and of self in relation to others in ways that enable the uniqueness and individuality of every human encounter to be more fully appreciated (Carper, 1978). Self-knowing may be nurtured through such processes as private meditation and journaling. It is communicated through personal stories that, in writing or in dialogue with others, create shared understandings of important elements about the therapeutic use of self in practice disciplines (Chinn & Kramer, 2004).

See **Patterns of Knowing.**

Phenomenological Reduction

Phenomenological reduction is an iterative recollective, reflective, introspective mental process that produces descriptions and interpretations of what life experiences are like for people. It involves *bracketing/epoche (recognizing one's own inner state and feelings/suspending presuppositions), retention (bringing to remembrance/keeping in mind the details of an experience), reflection (mentally reviewing/going over and over details), imaginative play (varying frames of reference/viewing the experience from different perspectives/searching for possible meanings), intuition (entertaining whatever enters awareness), and synthesis (writing/describing/interpreting).

See **Phenomenology.**

Phenomenology

As a field of concentration in philosophy, *phenomenology* is the study of the structures of experience as they present themselves to consciousness.

P

As a research tradition it is the investigation of what life experiences are like. Edmund Husserl (1859–1938) offered phenomenology as a response to and critique of positivist science's incapability of dealing with human experience because of its refusal to consider anything other than observable entities and objective reality as a focus of study. He argued for a return to 'the things themselves,' *essences* that constitute the pre-scientific world of human consciousness and perception, and introduced the concept of the *lifeworld (Lebenswelt),* or *lived experience,* as the natural world in which we live. The lifeworld is not readily accessible because it is made up of what we take for granted and therefore fail to explore. Husserl believed that the logic of what is taken for granted is the foundation and source upon which objective (positivist) science draws. Therefore, the task of phenomenology is to return to and to reexamine what we believe we already know and understand by reflectively bringing into awareness that which has been taken for granted.

The unifying thread in phenomenological research is that it always asks about the nature or meaning of the human experience—"What is it like?" However, it is unlikely that there will be a single unified approach to thinking about or 'doing' phenomenology.

Some major figures have inspired different styles and approaches to the study of phenomenology (e.g., Husserl's eidetic transcendentalism, Heidegger's hermeneutics, and Merleau-Ponty's existentialism). Researchers who cite their work should clarify how a particular perspective was used to guide their projects. Philosophical schools of thought are not 'procedurals' but there are texts on 'how to' conduct phenomenological research and models of many distinct styles. The differences among them make it important for researchers to describe and justify their methodological choices. Research styles may be more descriptive or more interpretive. The empirical-phenomenological psychology of the Duquesne school (Giorgi, Colaizzi, Fischer, and van Kaam) and the Husserlian transcendental phenomenology of Moustakas are examples of more descriptive styles. More interpretive styles include Heideggerian hermeneutics and the *human science pedagogy* of van Manen, an example of a combined approach (the German interpretive tradition of the Dilthey-Nohl School and the Dutch descriptive tradition of the Utrecht School). The most commonly cited phenomenological approaches to research in nursing are the diverse empirical-phenomenological approaches of the Duquesne school (Giorgi, Colaizzi, van Kaam) and the hermeneutic phenomenology of van Manen. For examples in the nursing literature, see Beck (2004), Carlsson, Dahlberg, Lützen, and Nystrom (2004), and Wilde (2002).

See **Bracketing, Intentionality, Intersubjectivity,** and **Phenomenological Reduction.**

Philosophical Inquiry

Philosophical inquiry in nursing is discursive (conversational) rather than investigative in nature. Its purpose is to critically debate issues that do not lend themselves to empirical analysis (although such discussions often stem from, lead to, or are intertwined with some combination of empirical/interpretive research activities). To illustrate, the International Philosophy of Nursing Society gives examples of types of philosophical issues in nursing for which their official journal provides a forum.

> What are the ends of nursing? . . . to promote health, prevent disease, promote well-being, enhance autonomy, relieve suffering, or some combination of these? . . . [And what are the] means by which these ends are to be met [i.e.] What kind of knowledge is needed in order to nurse? Practical, theoretical, aesthetic, moral, political, 'intuitive' or some other? In addition to these subject areas, [also encouraged are] critical discussions of the work of nurse theorists who have advanced philosophical claims [e.g.] Benner, Benner and Wrubel, Carper, Schrok, Watson, Parse [as well as philosophers who are] discussed with increasing frequency in nursing journals [e.g.] Heidegger, Husserl, Kuhn, Polanyi, Taylor, and MacIntyre (Edwards & Liaschenko, Eds., *Nursing Philosophy,* Home Page).

Following discussions pertaining to given topics may facilitate orientation to philosophical exchanges in the literature. For example, one could follow the arguments for grounding perspectives on nursing issues and inquiry in a philosophy of moderate realism (Kikuchi, 2003, 2004; Fraser & Strang, 2004). Or one could observe how the philosophy literature enters into debates about nursing, such as Benner's (2000) and Paley's (2002) different views on the relevance of Kant's philosophy for nursing practice.

Another way to gain familiarity with philosophical ways of thinking about nursing is to study the work of a particular nurse philosopher, such as Sally Gadow. Gadow has advanced existential advocacy as a moral framework for nursing practice. Her work appears in *Nursing Philosophy* and other journals (e.g., Gadow, 1995a, 1995b, 1999, 2000, 2003) and there are a number of articles both in praise and critique of the contributions of her philosophy to interpretive inquiry and to the nursing profession (e.g., Bishop & Scudder, 2003; McIntyre, 2003; Minicucci, Schmitt, Dombeck, & Williams, 2003; Paley, 2004).

Pilot Study

A *pilot study* is a preliminary 'try-out' of a research project with a small group of subjects who are similar to those to be recruited later. The purpose is to allow the researcher and any assistants to practice and evaluate the effectiveness of proposed data collection and analysis techniques.

Thus, problems with the methods can be detected and changes made when necessary before the large-scale project is launched. In addition, unexpected responses and findings may suggest new directions for the investigation or point out discrepancies that may need to be addressed.

Small-scale exploratory investigations are sometimes called pilot studies even though a larger study is not specifically planned at the time when they are undertaken. This may reflect the preliminary nature of the work, a need for baseline data, or the intention of the researcher to build research on the database generated by the pilot study. Many student theses, because of limitations of time and resources, could be identified as this sort of study.

The important thing when a pilot study precedes a planned study is to perform every step as it will be performed in the projected research. The main interest of the investigator is usually in the adequacy of data-collection instruments. 'Pretesting' of instruments and 'pilot studies' are sometimes discussed together in research texts as separate but related concepts. Pilot studies are more comprehensive, incorporating pretesting data-collection instruments along with a trial run of a study on a smaller scale that includes data analysis and reporting results.

For additional information on pilot studies, see Prescott and Soeken (1989). For examples of pilot studies in the nursing literature, see H. Li et al. (2003), Minardi and Blanchard (2004), and B. Parker, Steeves, Anderson, and Moran (2004).

Placebo

Placebo is a general term for a treatment that is very similar to the experimental treatment except that it lacks the essential ingredient that is of principal interest to the researcher.

The term comes from medical research, specifically from research on the effects of drugs such as aspirin or other analgesics. To pin down the effect of certain drugs it is essential to have at least two groups of subjects. The experimental group gets the pill (or liquid, or whatever) with the drug and the placebo group gets the pill (or liquid, or whatever) without the drug.

Example: If a researcher in nursing education wanted to test the effect of a particular film on the attitudes of nursing students toward abortion, she or he might randomly assign the students to two groups. One group would view the abortion film, and the other group would view a film with similar content but without any reference to abortion per se.

Point Estimation

Point estimation is a type of statistical inference in which a single sample statistic is claimed to be in some sense the 'best' estimate of the corresponding population parameter.

Example: Using the percentage of RNs in a sample to estimate the percentage of RNs in the population from which the sample was drawn.
See Inferential Statistics.

Population

A *population* is an entire set of people or hospitals or whatever that is of particular interest to the researcher.
See Inferential Statistics, Parameter, and Sampling.

Positive Relationship

A *positive relationship* between two variables, say X and Y, is one in which Y increases as X increases and Y decreases as X decreases, although not necessarily in perfect lockstep order. It is also called a direct relationship, but that term has a slightly different meaning in certain contexts such as path analysis in which the distinction is made between direct and indirect rather than between direct and inverse.

When the Pearson product-moment correlation coefficient is used to measure the relationship between two variables, a positive relationship is indicated by a number between 0 and +1.

Example: There is a positive relationship between height and weight for adult American females. That is, taller women tend to be heavier and shorter women tend to be lighter, but there are many exceptions. The Pearson r is approximately +.50.

Positivism

Positivism was the name given to a version of *strict empiricism* (the belief that experience as accessed through the senses is the only source of factual knowledge) developed by Auguste Comte (1798–1857) in 19th century France.

> Comte traced the development of human thought from its theological and metaphysical stages to its positive stage . . . characterized by systematic collection and correlation of observed facts and abandonment of unverifiable speculation about first causes or final ends [associated with the earlier stages] (Flew, 1979, p. 283).

He viewed science as the sole repository of all human knowledge and saw its role as making predictions and formulating laws based on observation. Over time there have been different versions of positivist/empiricist thinking that show responsiveness to internal shifts and external critiques while retaining and carrying over many basic beliefs into the present postpositivist/postempiricist era.

See Empiricism, Logical Empiricism, Logical Positivism, Postempiricism, and Postpositivism.

Postempiricism

Postempiricism is the term used after the abandonment of strict empiricism by modern empiricists whose views are more in line with current empirical philosophy of science perspectives. In philosophy, its use signals a focus on the nature and meaning of experience (e.g., the *radical empiricism* of William James or the *immediate empiricism* of John Dewey). In research, contemporary empiricism assumes that human responses can be identified, measured, and understood with some degree of predictability. "[T]here are two major tenets that serve as the foundation for all empirical thought: deductive reasoning [theory-linked and free of bias] and substantiation of theoretical claims [through systematic observation and standards of verification]" (Weiss, 1995, p. 16).

See **Empiricism** and **Postpositivism**.

Postmodernism

Postmodernism is a product of *modernism* as well as a response to *postmodernity*, (i.e., a cultural awakening to the limits of modernity). It is a broad term that refers to many characteristics that also have been applied to *modernism* (e.g., breaks with tradition, experimentation). However, as globalization with its trends in mass communication, mass marketing, and mass transportation makes the world appear 'smaller,' there is a sense that "[a]ll kinds of divisions and distinctions are evaporating. . . . Fragmentation takes the place of totality and completeness. Ambiguity reigns where there once was clarity. The old certainties vanish. . . ." (Crotty, 1998, pp. 193–194). Postmodernism involves exploration of that sense of fragmentation and ambiguity. However, it is a large 'umbrella term' that does not constitute a unified perspective or approach. Tarnas (1991) explains:

> . . . the postmodern mind may be viewed as an open-ended, indeterminate set of attitudes that has been shaped by a great diversity of intellectual and cultural currents; these range from pragmatism, existentialism, Marxism, and psychoanalysis to feminism, hermeneutics, deconstruction, and postempiricist philosophy of science, to cite only a few of the more prominent (p. 395).

In *Postmodern Nursing and Beyond,* J. Watson (1999) described this open-ended quality as an

> emerging . . . mindset [that] suggests there is no one Truth, but multiple truths; no one universally known reality that is defined by physical-material world. . . . [T]here is attention to valuing multiple meanings; acknowledgment of both physical and non-physical reality and phenomena . . . [and] open[ness] to ideas that include context, critiques, challenges, multiple interpretations, stories, narratives, text and search for meaning and wholeness" (p. 289).

She, therefore, encourages the nursing discipline to use this ontological shift in the ways in which life is now perceived to advance *transpersonal nursing* as a caring-healing model for the new millennium. For additional examples of references to postmodernism in nursing see N. Glass and Davis (2004), Glazer (2001), Holmes and Warelow (2000), Kendall, Hatton, Beckett, and Leo (2003), Reinhardt (2004), and Thompson (2002).

See **Modernism.**

Postpositivism

Postpositivism is a term that refers, historically, to the period following the failure of *logical positivism/logical empiricism* to locate the basis for all knowledge in sense experience. It is used both with reference to contemporary positivism and the pluralistic research environment in which it exists.

> [Contemporary positivism] is a less arrogant form of positivism . . . [that] talks of probability rather than certainty, claims a certain level of objectivity rather than absolute objectivity, and seeks to approximate the truth rather than aspiring to grasp it in its totality or essence (Crotty, 1998, p. 29).

Contemporary positivism reflects the position of Karl Popper (1902–1994), who emphasized falsifiability (the doctrine that we can only refute but never confirm) rather than verifiability in the testing of theories. The postpositive environment is one of greater variation in approaches to inquiry (e.g., constructivist, postempiricist, feminist, critical, phenomenological, hermeneutic, poststructuralist). ". . . [S]ome [individuals working within different traditions] reject positivism and the objectivism that informs it [while] . . . others remain within the positivist camp. . . ." (Crotty, p. 40). The postpositive theoretical perspective/paradigm has been described as objectivist in nature, deterministic in focus (a need to examine cause and effect), and reductionistic in intent (a need to reduce complex conceptualizations to discrete research questions and testable hypotheses). The emphasis is on operationalization, observation and measurement of objective reality, quantification, and verification (see Lincoln & Guba, 2000, and Creswell, 2003).

See **Logical Empiricism, Logical Positivism, Positivism,** and **Postempiricism.**

Poststructuralism

Poststructuralism, with its foundation in semiotics, is both a critique and a reinvention of the structuralist project. That is, it rejects structuralism but "retains structuralism's commitment to de Saussure's view that the meaning of words derives from their relationship to one another and not from any postulated relationship to non-linguistic reality" (Crotty, 1998, p. 203). Thus, the focus remains on language and the structure of discourse. Any phenomenon may be seen as one of many interrelated 'texts' (elements of structure). However, poststructuralism differs from the structuralist stance of the investigator 'standing outside of the text' and seeking to discover an objective universal underlying structure that can explain the relationships. The poststructuralist 'reader's' (investigator's) stance of engagement is such that it is impossible to step 'outside the text.' There also is no expectation of uncovering objective universal truths. Poststructuralist 'readings' are deconstructions that often are politically motivated to reveal multiple, opposing meanings that language may serve to obscure, with no one 'reading' being privileged over another. Beyond these generalities there is no unified poststructural 'approach' to inquiry. Well-known poststructuralist works are those of Jacques Derrida, Pierre Bourdieu, Michel Foucault, Roland Barthes, and Jacques Lacan. In the nursing literature, see Dickson (1990), Dzurec (2003), and Francis (2000).

See **Deconstruction, Semiotics,** and **Structuralism.**

Posttest

In experimental research a *posttest* is a test that is administered after the experiment has taken place.

See **Experiment.**

Postulate

A *postulate* is a type of proposition that is similar to an axiom and functions in the same way as an introductory premise in a formal logical reasoning process.

See **Theory, Proposition, Axiom,** and **Premise.**

Power

In a test of statistical significance, *power* is the probability of not making a Type II error, that is, the probability of correctly rejecting the null hypothesis when it is false. Cohen's (1988) book is the classic source for power and sample size determination.

See **Test of Significance.**

Pragmatism

Pragmatism is an American school of philosophy, historically associated with Kant's (1724–1804) *critique of practical reason* but better known through the work of Charles Sanders Peirce (1839–1914), William James (1842–1910), and John Dewey (1859–1952) as well as contemporary *neopragmatists* such as Richard Rorty and Richard Bernstein. There are different and conflicting versions of pragmatism. Generally, pragmatists are concerned about problems of 'truth' and 'meaning' in terms of their utility and consequences. Schwandt (2000) places neopragmatism under the umbrella of social *constructionism with other traditions whose view is that ". . . knowledge of what others are doing and saying always depends upon some background or context of other meanings, beliefs, values, practices, and so forth . . . [h]ence . . . understanding is interpretation all the way down" (p. 201). A notable way in which pragmatism has influenced the practice of qualitative inquiry is through pragmatist philosopher and social psychologist George Herbert Mead (1863–1931), on whose teachings and philosophy *symbolic interaction* is based. Symbolic interaction (a theory of communication) provides the philosophical foundation for ethnomethodology and grounded theory.

See **Ethnomethodology, Grounded Theory,** and **Symbolic Interaction.**

Praxis

Praxis is a term used by Marx (1818–1883) that refers to actual work, practice, or action in contrast to philosophical activity. It is associated with critical inquiry in the sense of translating the theory and rhetoric of social criticism into practice. However, the relationship between knowledge/theory and practice/action is close and intertwined. Therefore, for there to be any benefit, praxis must be understood as a complex activity involving (a) in theory—dialectical analyses and dialogues about models of praxis as well as (b) in practice—repeated cycles of action and critical reflection, with each repeating cycle reinforcing the fit between theory (awareness) and practice (autonomy). In the nursing literature, see Thorne and Hayes's (1997) excellent edited volume on *Nursing Praxis: Knowledge and Action,* which offers critical reflective analyses of the nature of knowledge in clinical practice, the application of theoretical ideas in practice, and ideas about the creation of new directions for emancipatory inquiry. See also Endo (2004) and Georges (2002).

See **Critical Theory** and **Participatory Action Research.**

Predictive Validity

Predictive validity is a type of criterion-related validity in which the data for the external criterion are obtained after the data for the instrument to be validated have been gathered.

See **Validity.**

Premise

A *premise* is an introductory propositional statement about the relationship between concepts in a theory. In mathematics and deductive logic, premises serve as the basis for forming a conclusion. Postulates and axioms are other types of premises.

See **Theory, Proposition, Postulate,** and **Axiom.**

Pretest

In experimental research a *pretest* is a test administered before the experiment is undertaken.

See **Experiment.**

Primary Source

A *primary source* is a source of original data, such as documents, memorabilia, or firsthand accounts. Primary sources are preferred over secondary sources because of the decreased potential for bias and distortion beyond the control of the researcher.

See **Secondary Source.**

Probability Sampling

Probability sampling is a type of sampling in which each object in the population has a known (but not necessarily equal) probability of being selected into the sample.

See **Sampling.**

Problem Solving

Problem solving is a process that uses research methods to meet program needs and to solve concrete problems. It tends to be cyclic in nature, involving assessment of a situation, setting goals and implementing a plan, evaluating the effectiveness of the plan, and making revisions, at which point the cycle repeats itself.

See **Evaluation Research.**

Proportion

Like a percentage, a *proportion* is a number that indicates part of a whole. It can take on any value between 0 (none) and 1 (all); it can easily be converted to a percentage by multiplying by 100 and affixing a % sign; and it is usually preferred for summarizing part/whole evidence in most statistical work.

Example: If a sample contains two males and three females, the proportion of females is 3 out of 5, or .60; the percentage of females is .60 × 100 = 60%.

See **Percentage.**

Proposition

A *proposition* is a statement about the relationships between concepts in a theory. It is a general label that includes postulates, premises, axioms, theorems, hypotheses, and laws. The terminology for different types of propositional statements varies according to the contexts in which they are used and the formal purposes served in logical deductive reasoning formats.

See **Theory.**

Prospective Study

Prospective study is synonymous with longitudinal study. It is a type of research in which one or more groups of subjects are followed across time and compared on one or more variables.

Williams, Oberst, and Bjorklund (1994) report the results of a prospective study of women with hip fractures.

See **Correlational Research** and **Longitudinal Study.**

Protected Health Information (PHI)

In the United States, *protected health information (PHI)* is any identifiable information relating to an individual's past or present health, including identifiers such as name, address, telephone number, medical record number, or any other number or code that could link the person to the information. HIPAA privacy regulations list all protected health information fields. Formal release of protected health information for research purposes must be obtained directly from research participants, their legal guardians, and/or health care proxies and, if medical record information is needed, via data use agreements with 'covered entities' (providers and agencies) that stipulate the conditions governing disclosure of limited data set information, as defined by HIPAA.

See **De-Identified/Limited Data Sets, HIPAA,** and **Informed Consent/Assent, and Permission.**

Protocol

When applied to research, the term *protocol* in its broadest sense refers to the overall action plan, which includes purpose and design, methods, and human subjects considerations to the extent that those apply. In a narrower sense, there may be standardized protocols used within a study (e.g., observation tools, interview guides, tests, and surveys) that represent agreed-upon ways to ensure consistency in communication about and collection/management of the data as well as the implementation of a treatment condition in intervention studies.

Purposive/Purposeful Sampling

Purposive/purposeful sampling is a type of nonprobability sampling in which the researcher selects only those subjects (e.g., persons, observations, material artifacts) that satisfy the needs of the study as they evolve across time. For example, a researcher may begin with *convenience sampling* (selection of any appropriate and readily available sources of information) or *snowball sampling* (obtaining new participants through the help of those who are already enrolled); but as the database grows, filling information needs, checking for *negative cases, developing a theory *(theoretical sampling)*, and seeking variation *(maximum variation sampling)* require more discriminating strategies.

See **Sampling** and **Theoretical Sampling.**

P

Q

Q Sort

A *Q sort* is a measurement strategy first introduced by the psychologist William Stephenson (1953) as a self-report technique for determining the relative relevance to an individual subject of a set of declarative statements. The subject is given a deck of cards, one statement per card, and is asked to sort those cards into several piles with designations ranging from 'most like me' to 'least like me.' The number of piles and the number of cards to be placed in each pile (but not which cards) are predetermined by the researcher and usually chosen so as to form a normal or near-normal frequency distribution.

Example: A nurse researcher interested in the reasons why people select nursing as a profession could prepare cards listing 16 reasons that might be given and ask each prospective student nurse to sort a deck of cards containing those reasons into five piles, with one card to be placed in the first pile (the subject's most compelling reason), four in the second pile, six in the third pile, four in the fourth pile, and one in the last pile (the least compelling reason).

For an example of a nursing research study that used a Q sort, see Puntillo and Weiss (1994).

Qualitative Research

Qualitative research is a broad cover term for many different research traditions concerned with the study of human experiences in and in relation to the natural contexts within which they occur for the purpose of understanding persons' responses and the meanings they bring to the experiences. Lincoln and Denzin (2000) describe qualitative research as a "humanistic commitment . . . to study the world always from the perspective of the gendered, historically situated, interacting individual" (p. 1047). In a field that cannot be described in terms of a single specific epistemological orientation, theoretical perspective, or methodology, these types of definitions provide a general introduction.

Epistemologies and theoretical perspectives: Qualitative researchers assume different epistemological stances that influence their work. Schwandt (2000) describes three 'epistemologies' that "vie for attention as potential justifications for doing qualitative inquiry" (p. 190). These include *interpretivism, *hermeneutics, and *constructionism. (Different authors may call some of these *theoretical perspectives to distinguish them from epistemological theories of knowledge, e.g., *objectivism, *subjectivism, *constructivism.) Another way to understand qualitative researchers' approaches to knowledge is by broader comparison of different *paradigms in relation to *epistemology, *ontology, and *methodology. See, for example, Guba and Lincoln (1994) and Lincoln and Guba (2000) for discussion of major issues confronting all paradigms, including *positivism, *postpositivism, *critical theory, *constructivism, and *participatory paradigms. Research-related discussions that focus on *methods and methodology involve many assumptions derived from these different ways of looking at the world and phenomena of interest to the researcher. These significant mindsets may or may not be recognized and/or acknowledged, but they can never be discounted.

Methodologies and Methods: Major research texts generally focus on the various methodologies (traditions) and methods (techniques) that characteristically fall under the broad umbrella of qualitative research. There is no single preferred way to distinguish methodologies. Most general texts cover the classical characteristics of *ethnography, *grounded theory, and *phenomenology. Creswell (1998) also discusses the qualitative *case study and *biography. Some texts discuss *hermeneutics. Theoretical perspectives or *ideologies, such as *critical theory or *feminism, that often are combined with qualitative research strategies as the 'vehicles' used to advance work in these areas, are sometimes mentioned as well. Texts that are devoted exclusively to one or another of these methodologies reveal much more complex pictures of the different types of research that make up the field. Many differences are sensitive to major philosophical and theoretical movements that have had a significant impact on approaches to science and scientific research. Some influences that are evident in the nursing literature are *functionalism, *structuralism, *poststructuralism, *modernism, and *postmodernism. The vastly different qualitative research methodologies employ a wide variety of methods, or techniques. Entire textbooks have been devoted to such topics as *fieldwork, *participant observation, and styles of *intensive indepth interviewing. These can be important and useful 'how to' guides. However, they are not the way to learn 'how to' be a qualitative researcher. Qualitative researchers have been mentored by other qualitative researchers and educated in their specialties from the top down, not from the bottom up.

See **Quantitative Research.**

Quality Assurance (QA)/Continuous Quality Improvement (CQI)

See **Evaluation Research.**

Quantitative Research

Although in isolation the term is not explicitly used very often, *quantitative research* is concerned with precise measurement, replicability, prediction, and control. It includes techniques and procedures such as standardized tests, random sampling and/or assignment, tests of statistical significance, and causal modeling. It may be preceded by descriptive pilot studies that are preliminary steps to a subsequent experimental or correlational study.

Quantitative studies have one or more of the following properties:

1. Adoption of the hypothesize-test-rehypothesize sequence that is characteristic of "the" scientific method.
2. Emphasis upon structured and objective measuring procedures.
3. Extensive use of numbers to reflect the measurements and to summarize the results.
4. An emphasis on causality.

Path analysis, treated elsewhere in this dictionary, is a prototypical quantitative research approach. A model regarding one possible state of the world is postulated, tested, and (if warranted) revised. Data for testing the model are usually based on objective measuring instruments. The numbers yielded by those instruments are analyzed to produce other numbers that assist the researcher in deciding which hypotheses in the model to accept and which to reject.

The label of quantitative research is not a good one, though, because it is difficult to call to mind any study that does not or could not involve some quantification. When quantitative research is contrasted with qualitative research (an equally problematic cover term), the label has come to stand for an orientation characterized by the insistence that science can only deal with observable phenomena and that systematically controlled and regulated observation and experiment will reveal general laws that demonstrate the relationships between phenomena. The orientation comes from a belief that the social and human sciences can be scientific in the same way as mathematics or physics, and thus there is a distinct preference for measurement and quantification, as well as a tendency to deduce explanations of social phenomena that avoid focusing on or dealing with human subjectivity—perceptions, intentions, motives. Therefore, it is more accurate to regard differences between quantitative and qualitative research as differences in research purpose and orientation than it is to differentiate between such studies on the basis of preferred methods, for example, whether they involve description or quantification. Quantitative approaches have descriptive aspects and qualitative approaches may use counts, measurement techniques, and statistical analyses. Methods or techniques should not be the basis for the ways in which research is thought about or labeled.

Some textbooks in nursing research contain discussions of both qualitative research and quantitative research. Some are concerned solely with qualitative research. One book that is dedicated to quantitative nursing research only is Knapp (1998).

See **Qualitative Research.**

Quasi-Experiment

A *quasi-experiment* is an experiment that has manipulation and some controls but lacks random assignment of individual subjects to the treatment conditions.

True experiments with random assignment are thought to provide the most powerful tests of research hypotheses concerned with cause-and-effect relationships, because of the extent to which extraneous influences may be controlled. There are many instances, however, when a true experiment is not feasible; that is, random assignment cannot be carried out. For such quasi-experiments serious consideration must be given to other factors that might possibly have affected the outcome of the study. These alternative explanations are called 'threats to internal validity.' Quasi-experimental designs attempt to compensate for the absence of randomization in various ways. (See Campbell & Stanley, 1966, and Cook & Campbell, 1979, for descriptions of a number of quasi-experimental designs.) In spite of their limitations, quasi-experiments are frequently more practical in nursing research that takes place in settings less amenable to full experimental control.

Some authors use the term quasi-experiment very broadly to denote any 'experiment-like' study that involves the comparison of two or more groups, with or without the actual manipulation of the principal independent variable by the researcher.

Example: Since it is at best awkward to randomly assign individual Alzheimer's patients to receive Drug A or Drug B, the investigator interested in determining the relative effectiveness of the two drugs might choose to give Drug A to patients in one health care facility and to give Drug B to patients in another health care facility, and use some sort of statistical procedure to adjust the data to take into account the fact that the groups may not have been equivalent at the beginning of the experiment. Note, however, that any sort of statistical control is inferior to the direct control provided by the random assignment that is characteristic of a true experiment.

Berkhout, Boumans, Van Breukelen, Abu-Saad, and Nijhuis (2004) used a quasi-experimental design in their study of resident-oriented care in nursing homes.

Quota Sampling

Quota sampling is a type of nonprobability sampling in which, as the term implies, sampling continues until certain quotas are filled. It is used quite frequently in certain kinds of opinion polls that attempt to sample so many women, so many men, so many Whites, so many Blacks, and so forth. The typical pollster may be asked to walk down a city block and find a Black female, a male over 35 years of age, and so forth.

Quota sampling should not be confused with stratified random sampling, which is a type of probability sampling.

See **Sampling.**

Q

R

Random Assignment

Random assignment is a means of control in a true experiment. Individual subjects are allocated to the treatment conditions in such a way that chance and chance alone determines which subjects receive which treatments.

Groups to which subjects are randomly assigned may be judged to be equal in a statistical sense at the beginning of the experiment, although they may not actually be equal in every respect. As the sizes of the groups increase, so does the probability that they are similar, if random assignment has been carried out properly. Some methodologists suggest coupling simple random assignment with a technique called "minimization" in order to achieve better balance across treatment conditions with respect to possibly confounding variables—see, for example, Zeller et al. (1997).

Random assignment may be accomplished by using coins, cards, tables of random numbers, or other devices that eliminate any biases that an investigator may have, consciously or unconsciously, in allocating subjects to treatment conditions.

Example: A nurse physiologist carrying out basic research on rat endocrinology might randomly assign half of a sample of rats to receive an injection of one type of hormone and the other half to receive an injection of a second type of hormone in order to study the comparative effects of the two types of hormones on feeding behavior.

Random Sampling

Random sampling is a type of sampling in which chance and chance alone determines which subjects in a population are drawn into a research sample. The purpose of random sampling is to provide a statistical basis for generalizing the results of the research from the sample actually employed to the larger population of interest.

144

Simple random sampling is a type of random sampling in which every subject in the population has an *equal* chance of being drawn into the sample. *Stratified* random sampling necessitates the division of the population into two or more subpopulations called strata and taking a random sample from each stratum.

Just as for random assignment, devices such as coins, cards, or a table of random numbers can be used to draw the sample. But it is essential to keep in mind that random sampling and random assignment are <u>not</u> the same thing.

The terms *random sampling* and *probability sampling* are often used interchangeably.

Example: In attempting to estimate the percentage of registered nurses who smoke cigarettes, a researcher might obtain a directory of all registered nurses in a particular state and use a table of random numbers to select the sample to whom a self-report questionnaire could be mailed.

Randomized Clinical Trial (RCT)

A randomized clinical trial is the "gold standard" for investigating causality in intervention research.

See **Clinical Trial.**

Range

The *range* of a set of data for a variable is the difference between the lowest value and the highest value for the variable.

Rapid Assessment Process/Rapid Appraisal

Rapid assessment process (RAP) or rapid appraisal (RA) is an approach for obtaining preliminary sociocultural understanding of situations prior to the development of programs or interventions. It also may be used for evaluation purposes. In the mid-1970s, the concept of *rapid appraisal (RA)* caught researchers' attention in connection with *rapid rural appraisal (RRA)* protocols used to plan, execute, and evaluate third world farming system development projects (Beebe, 1995). In the practice of applied anthropology it is used in situation-specific ways, for example, the design, implementation, and evaluation of public health and nutrition intervention programs, or *rapid marketing appraisal (RMA)* in the evaluation of local economies (e.g., agricultural markets, forestry). Authors use different words for the letter 'P' in the *RAP* acronym (e.g., *program, procedures, practice, protocol*). However, techniques are consistent despite terminological variations (Beebe, 2001).

RAP/RA approaches substitute intensive team interaction over a short period of time (weeks) for the longer periods of intense fieldwork (years) that is a traditional hallmark of anthropological/ethnographic studies.

RAP teams are not large, but they should contain a mix of *insiders* (members of the host culture or identified *stakeholders) and *outsiders* (guest advisors/researchers) plus at least one member with expertise in qualitative fieldwork methods. All team members are involved in informal group interviews conducted by at least two members, in which local participants/identified stakeholders are encouraged and given time to tell their stories and share their insights. An iterative process of data analysis directs additional data collection. The aim is to obtain the fullest possible understanding of the situation from insiders' perspectives. Overall, the success of RAP outcomes is dependent on the quality of team interaction. After the team leaves the field, *insider* team members maintain communication about project results, community/stakeholder responses, and outstanding or resultant issues.

It is important to understand that a RAP study is <u>not</u> a 'mini-ethnography.' Rather, it is a pragmatic alternative to ethnographic studies when the need for results is immediate. It cannot provide the holistic cultural portraits and interpretive insights that are characteristic of traditional *ethnography. But, by adapting some of the techniques that ethnographers use to a team-based approach and applying them in a given situation, it can generate important understandings that may inform public policy and help to lay the groundwork for larger community service or research initiatives. See Beebe (2001).

Ratio Scale

A *ratio scale* is a level of scientific measurement characterized by the existence of a unit of measurement and a "real" zero point that is indicative of absence of the construct being measured. The only permissible transformations of ratio scales are those of the restricted linear form $Y = bX$.

Example: Force (in dynes, say) is a typical example of a ratio scale. A "score" of zero on that variable means no force. There is nothing special about the dyne, however; any multiplicative transformation to some other convenient unit is perfectly acceptable.

See Scale.

Realism

Realism is the ontological assumption that there are 'objects' in the universe that exist independent of human knowledge or awareness of them. These are what *objectivist* approaches to inquiry (see *objectivism*) seek to make sense of. However, there are many different realist philosophies, only some of which will be mentioned here. The 'naïve realism' of *positivism assumed a knowable 'real' reality 'out there' ruled by natural laws and accessible through the human senses. The 'critical realism' of *postpositivism, in contrast, assumes a 'real' reality with the proviso that it can only be known imperfectly and probabilistically. (See Guba & Lincoln, 1994; Lincoln & Guba, 2000.) The relationship of *realism* to qualitative inquiry (see *subjectivism* and* constructivism*) is more complex. For example, though both are epistemologically subjectivist, the *relativism of constructivist approaches contrasts with the 'historical realism' of *critical theory as described by Guba and Lincoln. Historical realism assumes that a reality shaped over time by combinations of "social, political, cultural, economic, ethnic, and gender factors and then crystallized (reified) into a series of structures that are now (inappropriately) taken as 'real' . . . [is] for all practical purposes . . . [an apprehensible] historical reality" (p. 110). For another sense of the term, see Van Maanen's (1988) classic *Tales of the Field* and the literature on *representation in qualitative research which describe the 'realist' posture as one that presents observed/perceived reality in a factual authoritative manner. Many interpretive practices challenge this reporting style; but, pragmatically, there is little disagreement that 'objects' (e.g., persons, events, social structures) exist in many ways independent from the investigator. The objection to *realism* here has been of 'naïve realism's' view of 'real' reality and the researcher's relationship (separation of subject and object) to it. Realism is opposed by idealism.

See **Idealism** and **Ontology.**

Receiver Operating Characteristic Curve

A *receiver operating characteristic (ROC) curve* has nothing to do with receiving, operating, or characterizing, but is a device for displaying sensitivity and specificity data. It can also be used to depict the difference between two groups on an ordinal scale, in which case it is sometimes called an 'ordinal dominance' curve.

For an interesting example of the use of an ROC curve, see S. J. Bennett et al. (2003).

Recursive Model

In path analysis and structural equation modeling a recursive model is one that admits only one-way (i.e., not reciprocal) causation.

See **Path Analysis** and **Structural Equation Modeling.**

Reductionism

In philosophy, *reductionism* refers to theories that support the belief that complex phenomena can be reduced to (i.e., explained by) a smaller number of fundamental parts that make up the larger whole. This contrasts with theories that support *holism,* which holds that "whole" entities or collectivities are different than the sum of their individual parts. In research, methodologies that isolate and operationalize variables to

R

study their nature, relationships, and effects on one another, in terms of causality, are necessarily reductionistic. However, because *reductionistic* has been used as a pejorative, researchers employing these procedures tend not to use the term in relation to their work.

See **Holism** and **Determinism.**

Reflexivity

In qualitative research, the term *reflexivity* refers to a continual process of critical self-reflection on one's personal biases, preconceived notions, assumptions, theoretical predispositions, and ideological commitments. Researchers are encouraged to record their personal responses, reactions, and insights into their own feelings and behaviors in field diaries. These recordings are data, given that researchers cannot separate themselves from the social setting and phenomena that are the objects of study. Thus, reflexivity informs the analysis. At the same time, these procedures constitute one way to establish bias control and maintain the accuracy and completeness (i.e., validity) of field observations.

See **Bias** and **Validity.**

Regression Analysis

Regression analysis is a statistical procedure for studying the relationships between variables and determining the extent to which independent variables, individually and collectively, can predict and/or explain some dependent variable.

The focus of the regression analysis may be any or all of the following:

1. The determination of a mathematical model that best fits the data. This model is in the form of a linear regression equation, $Y = a+b_1X_1+b_2X_2+ \ldots +b_pX_p$, where Y is the dependent variable, the Xs are the independent variables, a is the intercept, the bs are the regression slopes, and p is the number of independent variables.
2. The determination of how well the model fits the data.
3. The determination of the statistical significance of the fit.

Those who emphasize the regression equation itself are concerned primarily with the regression coefficients—the intercept *(a)* and the slopes (the bs). (The intercept is equal to zero and the bs are called beta weights if the regression equation is in standardized form.) Those who concentrate on how well the equation fits the data emphasize correlation coefficients or their squares, which give some indication of the extent to which the independent and dependent variables vary together. Those who pursue the statistical significance of the intercept, the slopes, the squares of the correlation coefficients, and so forth are attempting to ascertain whether or not the fit of the equation to sample data could be attributable to chance alone.

There are several types of regression analyses: simultaneous, hierarchical, stepwise, and logistic. These are defined in separate entries in this dictionary.

Unfortunately, there is little or no agreement regarding what sort of information should be reported in an article concerning the results of a regression analysis. Knapp (1994) tried to remedy that situation.

The variables in a regression analysis are usually interval or ratio scales, but dichotomies can also be used as independent variables if they have been generated by dummy coding or other ways of redefining nominal or ordinal variables.

Example: In nursing education research, interest might center on the predictability of grade point average in a master's degree program *(Y)* by some combination of undergraduate grade point average (X_1), the quantitative score on the Graduate Record Examination (X_2), and the verbal score on that exam (X_3). Polit and Beck (2004, pp. 514–517) use this example in their discussion of multiple regression analysis, that is, regression analysis for which there is more than one independent variable. Three very popular multiple regression analysis texts are Darlington (1990), Pedhazur (1997), and Cohen, Cohen, West, and Aiken (2003).

R

Relative Risk
See **Risk.**

Relativism
Relativism is the ontological assumption that there is nothing about human existence that is universally true. There are many types of 'relativism' that usually are some sort of reaction against failure to take history, culture, and political and/or social environments into account when determining what is true, good, bad, right, or wrong about something. From this perspective, a description/interpretation of a phenomenon is not a mirror image of it but a report of how it is viewed and meaningfully constructed by certain persons or a given group of persons. Constructivism is a relativist *epistemology. Relativism is sometimes seen as the opposite of *objectivism. In *Beyond Objectivism and Relativism,* Bernstein (1983) discusses the strong points of both positions before setting out his own hermeneutical position, drawing on the philosophy of Gadamer (1900–2002).

See **Constructivism/Constructionism** and **Ontology.**

Reliability
Reliability is a technical term that has several meanings. As far as measurement is concerned, an instrument is called reliable if it produces *consistent* measures from time to time, from measurer to measurer, and so forth. But the term is also used in statistical analysis (a sample statistic is

reliable if it doesn't vary much from sample to sample) and in engineering (a piece of equipment is reliable if it is unlikely to break down while it is being used). To make matters even more confusing, lay people use the term *reliability* in the same sense that the term *validity* (another very important measurement concept) is used by social scientists, for example, "The custodian is very reliable."

The reliability of a measuring instrument is usually determined by one or more of the following procedures:

1. Parallel forms (equivalence)—for tests that have two equivalent forms, say A and B, scores on Form A are compared with scores on Form B.

2. Test-retest (stability)—the same persons are measured on two separate occasions and the Time 1 scores are compared with the Time 2 scores.

3. Split halves (internal consistency)—the test is administered just once but for scoring purposes the scores on half of the test are correlated with the scores on the other half of the test (usually the odd-numbered questions vs. the even-numbered questions) and the Spearman-Brown formula is used to estimate the reliability of the entire test.

4. Coefficient alpha (internal consistency)—again the test is administered just once and a special formula is used to estimate reliability.

Researchers are often also interested in interrater reliability, referring to a variety of techniques for determining the reliability of the *scoring* of a test (it is actually the *objectivity* of measurement with which such techniques are concerned).

There are competing theories regarding the reliability of measuring instruments, the most well-known being the classical test theory of true scores and obtained scores (Knapp, 2005). A true score on a variable is the measurement that a person *deserves* to get and would get if the instrumentation were perfectly reliable. An obtained score is the measurement that a person *does* get; it may or may not be equal to the corresponding true score. The difference between a person's obtained score and the corresponding true score is called an error score (or simply, an error). The errors are assumed to be *random* and not systematic.

It is essential to understand that the distinction between a true score and an obtained score is a matter of reliability and not validity (Knapp, 1985). The measuring instrument may or may not be a valid device for operationalizing the construct of interest. That is a separate issue. A person's obtained score may be very close to his or her true score on a valid test or on an invalid test. It could also be very different from the true score for both kinds of tests.

Individual true scores are of course always unknown. But by making certain reasonable assumptions, several interesting results can be demonstrated regarding groups of true scores. For example, the mean true score is equal to the mean obtained score and the correlation between the true scores on one test and the true scores on another test is equal to the correlation between the obtained scores divided by the square root of the product of the reliability coefficients (the so-called correction for attenuation).

Nursing researchers with a biophysiological bent tend to take a slightly different, yet still 'quantitative' approach to reliability (see Engstrom, 1988; and DeKeyser & Pugh, 1990).

Example: If one were interested in determining the reliability of a test such as the Miller Analogies Test (a test often used for admission to graduate study), any or all of the above methods might be appropriate. The test does have several parallel forms; stability of scores from one time to the next might be of interest. It consists of 100 items for which split halves and/or coefficient alpha analysis might be desired. Finally, although it is allegedly perfectly objective because it can be machine scored, it might be interesting to see if two scorers using the same scoring key would have 100% agreement.

Lincoln and Guba (1985) have described *dependability* as the qualitative concept that parallels *reliability*. Dependability is demonstrated by a research process that is carefully documented to provide evidence of how conclusions were reached and whether, under similar circumstances, another researcher might expect to obtain similar findings (i.e., the concept of the *audit trail*).

See **Audit Trail** and **Trustworthiness Criteria.**

Repeated-Measures Design

A *repeated-measures design* is a type of experimental design in which subjects are exposed to all of the treatments, in randomized order.

For a recent nursing research example, see Maxton, Justin, and Gillies (2004).

See **Experiment.**

Replication

The term *replication* has two different, though related, meanings in scientific research. *Within* an experimental study, especially those studies involving repeated-measures designs, each 'subject' (person, rat, hospital, etc.) is called a replication, or replicate. However, the more common usage is *across* studies, where a second study that is carried out on the same research problem is called a replication of the first study.

In that second sense of the term, replication studies have been both downplayed and encouraged. A doctoral student who would like to see if the results of X's study would be repeatable for a different sample of patients might be criticized for proposing an investigation that is "only" a replication of X's work. On the other hand, there is a constant cry for such studies because X's results might very well be unique to the particular situation that X chose to look at. (Perhaps the master's thesis is the ideal vehicle for replication studies?)

It is also not clear exactly what replication means in this second sense of the term. Must the second study duplicate every single aspect of the first study except one (e.g., the sample of subjects)? Or is it a replication study if it is merely an investigation of the same general research topic in a similar manner?

Example: A study of the effect of cigarette smoking on lung cancer in a highly industrialized environment would have to be replicated at least once in a pollution-free rural environment to get a better feel for whether the incidence of the cancer is linked with the cigarette smoking, with the pollution, or with some complicated confounding of the two.

Representation

Representation is part of the analytic process in qualitative research that raises the issue of providing a truthful portrayal of what the data represent (e.g., an *essence of an experience, a cultural portrait, a process individuals go through) that will be meaningful to the intended audience. There are many representational styles, and although there are standards and conventions, reporting is not standardized or formulaic. The issue for researchers is to be true to the data in terms of their validity while recognizing that an interpretation is not a mirror image of reality.

> The crisis of representation [is forever questioning]: Who is the Other? Can we ever hope to speak authentically of the experience of the Other, or an Other? And if not, how do we create a . . . science that includes the Other? (Lincoln & Denzin, 2000, p. 1050).

Validity and authenticity are central to the narrative and political issues attendant on attempts to 'voice' others' *worldviews and concerns.

A critical view of representation questions the 'rights of representation' in terms of who may speak for another. Researchers who engage in participatory research where study participants are viewed as 'co-investigators' see this as a way to move toward more empowering communally generated knowledge. They describe "conjoint representations" where "the line between researcher and subject is blurred, and control over representation is increasingly shared" . . . [Experimental methodologies are part of this movement, as in the example of] "distributed representation" [where the researcher] "attempts . . . to set in motion an array of different voices in dialogical relationship" (Gergen & Gergen, 2000, p. 1035).

There are many scholarly debates and volumes written about representation in the field of qualitative inquiry. However, Lincoln and Denzin (2000) suggest that the "short answer" to questions posed about ever hoping to speak authentically of the experience of the other "is that we move to including the Other in the larger research processes that we have developed," which will mean different things in different design contexts (p. 1050).

See **Voice.**

Research

Research is a systematic process of investigation, the general purpose of which is to contribute to the body of knowledge that shapes and guides academic and/or practice disciplines. Thus, the purpose of clinical nursing research is to improve the health, care, and quality of life of individuals, families, and communities through inquiries that address relevant professional practice issues. We take the position here that support for a pluralistic stance regarding the theoretical perspectives and methodological approaches used in research is vital for integrated knowledge development in nursing (see entry for *patterns of knowing*) as well as for nursing's continued active participation in an increasingly diverse and complex interdisciplinary research environment.

A necessary condition for this type of pluralism is an understanding of the processes that produce different approaches to research. The following quote is Crotty's (1998) description of four interrelated elements of any research process.

- *methods:* the techniques or procedures used to gather and analyse data related to some research question or hypothesis.
- *methodology:* the strategy, plan of action, process or design lying behind the choice and use of particular methods and linking the choice and use of methods to the desired outcomes.
- *theoretical perspective:* the philosophical stance informing the methodology and thus providing a context for the process and grounding its logic and criteria.
- *epistemology:* the theory of knowledge embedded in the theoretical perspective and thereby in the methodology (Crotty, 1998, p. 3).

Reversing the order of these elements illustrates how epistemology and theoretical perspectives inform decisions about what will be studied, how it will be studied, and how the results of the research will be used and interpreted.

Research may be categorized by type. For example, _basic/fundamental research_ primarily is concerned with developing the knowledge base and extending theory in academic and/or practice disciplines. In contrast to applied research, findings cannot always be applied directly to practice. However, their abstract, theoretical nature makes them generalizable to a variety of situations, and their utility may be tested through applied research. _Applied research_ is concerned with using knowledge generated by an investigation to develop practical approaches to problematic situations in a field or discipline. Findings may be less generalizable than those of basic research because of the focus on specific problems. However, there is complementarity between the two approaches when the usefulness of new knowledge produced by basic research is tested by applied research. *_Translational research_ is a subset of applied research that involves the translation of basic research knowledge into direct applications. *_Evaluation research_ refers to activities that use research methods and a *problem-solving process to meet program or practice needs. Quality assurance/continuous quality improvement studies are examples of evaluation research.

Research Utilization

Research utilization (RU) is a term that sometimes is used interchangeably with _evidence-based practice (EBP)_. However, they are two historically different movements, and despite overlaps, evidence-based practice is the broader of the two concepts. Ciliska, DiCenso, Melnyk, and Stetler (2005) helpfully distinguish between RU and EBP, explaining that

> [r]esearch utilization is the use of research knowledge, often based on a single study, in clinical practice, whereas EBP involves a larger skill set that takes into consideration all of the following factors: best evidence from a thorough search and critical appraisal of all relevant studies, context, healthcare resources, practitioner skills, patient status and circumstances, patient preferences and values. [They discuss] selected models developed to advance research utilization and EBP (p. 187).

There is a further connotation that may be associated with the concept of research utilization. That connotation is that RU is an institutional enterprise, in contrast to EBP, which can be institutional or individual. See also Olade's (2004) review of literature on research utilization for evidence-based practice in health care delivery and Veeramah's (2004) study that identifies barriers to RU for graduate nurses and midwives.

Retrospective Study

A _retrospective study_ is a type of correlational research in which a search is made, after the fact, for one or more independent variables that are potential causes of the dependent variable(s). Such studies are called case-control studies by epidemiologists.

See **Case-Control Study** and **Correlational Research.**

Risk

One of the key concepts in epidemiological research is the matter of *risk*. Risks are expressed in terms of proportions or percentages, and are interpreted as probabilities.

For example, if 10 out of 100 people who smoke cigarettes get lung cancer, the risk of lung cancer for cigarette smokers is $10/100 = 1/10 = 10\%$. Some other risk measures are:

Relative risk is the risk for one group divided by the risk for another group. For example, if 2 out of 100 people who don't smoke cigarettes get lung cancer, their risk is $2/100 = 1/50 = 2\%$, and their relative risk compared to smokers is $2\%/10\% = 1/5$; that is, they are one-fifth as likely to get lung cancer. Or, putting it the other way around, the relative risk for smokers compared to nonsmokers is $10\%/2\% = 5$; that is, smokers are five times as likely to get lung cancer.

Attributable risk is the difference between two risks (rather than their quotient). For the example just given, the attributable risk is $10\% - 2\% = 8\%$. Although the word *attributable* is used, the difference may or may not be <u>caused</u> by the smoking.

There are a few other risk-type terms that are occasionally encountered in the evidence-based practice (EBP) literature. See the extensive glossary for the Cochrane Collaboration and the brief glossary in the EBP 'bible' written by Sackett, Straus, Richardson, Rosenberg, and Haynes (2000).

See **Epidemiological Research.**

R

S

Sample

A *sample* is a subset of a population. It is often studied in preference to the entire population because of practical considerations such as cost and availability.

  See **Inferential Statistics** and **Sampling.**

Sampling

Sampling is the process of selecting a subset of objects from a larger set (population) of objects. Except for certain kinds of surveys, sampling tends to receive short shrift in nursing research. Yet from a scientific point of view it is hard to imagine anything more important than the representativeness of the sample upon which an investigation has been based.

  Research samples can be probability samples or nonprobability samples, the former always being the more desirable in quantitative research. In probability sampling every object in the population of interest has a *known* probability of being drawn into the sample. A simple random sample is one for which the probability of selection of an object is *equal* to that for every other object. (The selection of a given object must also be independent of the selection of another object.)

  But there are at least two other kinds of probability sampling. The first is stratified random sampling, whereby the population is divided into two or more subpopulations, or *strata,* and a simple random sample is selected from each *stratum.* In this way one can ensure that the sample is representative of the population with respect to at least one variable, namely the variable (sex, race, etc.) that produced the strata. For simple random sampling without stratification the sample is only *likely* to be representative. (A simple random sample of 25 people drawn from a large population that is 50% male and 50% female may, but probably will not, consist of all same-sex members.)

Another type of probability sampling is multistage cluster sampling. At the first stage, 10 large cities might be drawn at random; at the second stage, 2 hospitals might be drawn at random from each of the 10 cities; finally, all nurses at each of those 20 hospitals might be asked to participate in the research. This is quite different from having a 'sampling frame' (list) of nurses and drawing a simple random sample of nurses from that sampling frame. The analysis of the data for the former case is also different (and more complicated) because between-hospital and between-city variation must be taken into account as well as between-nurse variation.

Nonprobability sampling includes all sampling procedures (quota sampling, volunteer sampling, 'convenience' sampling, 'snowball' sampling, 'purposive' sampling) where chance plays no role in the determination of the actual constitution of the sample.

The following diagram may be helpful in distinguishing between probability and nonprobability sampling, and among their various subtypes:

Sampling:	Probability	Nonprobability
	Simple	Quota
	Stratified	Volunteer
	Cluster	Convenience
		Snowball
		Purposive

One type of sampling that could fall under either heading is systematic sampling, that is, sampling of 'every kth' object. If the starting point in sampling from a list is chosen at random, there is a probabilistic aspect. If not, that kind of sampling falls into the nonprobability category.

It is essential to distinguish among the terms *target population, sampled population, drawn sample,* and *responding sample.* The target population is the population that the researcher really cares about; it may or may not coincide with the population that is actually sampled. There may also be some attrition between the sample drawn and the responding sample. Some surveys regarding very sensitive topics such as attitudes toward abortion have extremely low response rates. The investigator may have drawn the sample at random from some accessible population, but it is the generalization from responding sample to target population that is of usual interest. Strictly speaking, statistical inference is only appropriate for generalizing from the drawn sample to the sampled population.

Finally, there is the matter of sample size. The extreme cases are easy. If you cannot afford to be wrong at all when generalizing from sample to population, you must take the whole population. If you don't mind being very wrong, take one object. But between $n = 1$ and $n =$ all, it depends on *how far wrong* you can afford to be, the assumed homogeneity of the population, the number of variables, and many other things. Fortunately there exist formulas and tables (e.g., Cohen, 1988) to help out.

Example: In a survey of nurses' smoking behavior, simple random sampling of the most recent American Nurses Association (ANA) directory should provide a reasonably representative 'snapshot' of such behavior by professional nurses (to the extent to which the directory mirrors the profession), particularly if the sample size is large (say 1,000 or so), the response rate is good, and the questions are straightforward.

In qualitative research, sampling is *purposive,* that is, there is a deliberate selection of study subjects, objects, or events to meet the needs of the research. Morse (1998b) explains, "the sample *must* be biased" toward informants who, in the researcher's judgment, will do the best job of representing the phenomenon of interest (p. 734). Sample size is characteristically determined by the principle of *saturation, for example, when the quality of the data meets study needs (theoretical saturation) and when informational categories and dimensions are 'saturated' to the extent that further sampling and data gathering strategies suggest no new directions and yield no new understandings (informational redundancy). However, samples may be "too small . . . [precluding the understanding of a phenomenon because] "[i]mpatience, and a priori commitment to what will be seen, or a disinclination to see any more may incline researchers to stop sampling prematurely" (Sandelowski, 1995, pp. 179–180). Samples also may be too large.

> An adequate sample size in qualitative research is one that permits—by virtue of not being too large—the deep, case-oriented analysis that is a hallmark of all qualitative inquiry, and that results in—by virtue of not being too small—a new and richly textured understanding of experience (Sandelowski, p. 183).

Morse (2000) discusses factors that should be considered when estimating sample size, including the specific qualitative method and study design that is being used, the scope of the study, the nature of the topic, the quality of the data, and the use of shadowed data.

See **Purposive/Purposeful Sampling.**

Sampling Distribution

A *sampling distribution* is a frequency distribution such as *t*, *F*, or chi-square that is used for making statistical inferences from samples to populations.

See **Inferential Statistics.**

Saturation

Saturation in qualitative research is a sense of closure that occurs when data collection ceases to provide new information and when relationships and patterns in the data are fully developed (data saturation). Theoretical saturation is accompanied by personal saturation as the researcher concludes that the aims of the analysis have been carried out as far as possible. However, the dangers of premature closure are very real, and researchers need to be sure that they have sampled broadly and appropriately, analyzed data carefully, pursued *negative cases, and completely understood all of the properties and dimensions of informational categories and their relationships (saturation of categories). For researchers whose research programs form a trajectory across a number of individual studies, saturation is always conditional since their 'research' is conceived as ongoing. Charmaz (2000) observes:

> The data in works claiming to be grounded theory pieces range from a handful of cases to sustained field research. The latter more likely fulfills the criterion of saturation and, moreover, has the resonance of intimate familiarity with the studied world (p. 520).

Scale

As the term is most often used in social measurement, a *scale* is a group of items that 'hang together.' The term is also used in conjunction with the modifiers 'nominal,' 'ordinal,' 'interval,' and 'ratio' to provide one way of classifying variables. And there are bathroom scales for measuring weight, Fahrenheit and centigrade (Celsius) scales for measuring temperature, and so forth.

To determine the extent to which certain test items constitute a scale, a variety of techniques is available. The two most popular procedures are factor analysis and scalogram analysis. In the former procedure all of the inter-item correlations are obtained and subjected to a complicated statistical analysis that generates one or more 'underlying' factors. Those items that have high 'loadings' on the same factor go together to make up a scale (or perhaps a subscale). Scalogram analysis is similar, but the emphasis is on the coefficient of reproducibility, which is a measure of how well a group of items approximates what is called a Guttman scale (see separate entry).

A nominal scale is a variable such as religious affiliation for which measurement consists merely in designating a qualitative category (Catholic, Protestant, etc.) into which a person falls. An ordinal scale is a bit more precise and consists of a set of *ordered* categories (e.g., the traditional 'strongly agree,' 'agree,' 'undecided,' 'disagree,' 'strongly disagree' categories used in Likert scales). An interval scale, best exemplified by something like outdoor temperature in degrees centigrade (Celsius), is one step higher because the categories (–10, 0, +20, etc.) are not only ordered, but there is a meaningful unit (the degree) that is constant throughout the scale. A ratio scale is the highest level of measurement,

S

and for such scales (e.g., physical force measured in dynes) there is a 'real' zero point in addition to ordered categories with a constant unit. (The zero point for physical force is *no force,* whereas the zero point in degrees Celsius for outdoor temperatures is *not* no temperature; it is simply that rather arbitrary point at which water becomes ice.) The terms *nominal scale, ordinal scale, interval scale,* and *ratio scale* are due to Stevens (1946).

Polit and Beck (2004) include several sections in their text that deal with scales in all of the above senses.

Example: A Toledo self-balancing *scale* yields weights that constitute data for a ratio *scale.*

Science

Science is both the process and the outcome of the systematic pursuit of knowledge as defined by a community of scholars. However, there is not agreement among scholars regarding what science is and which disciplines or disciplinary fields may claim to be scientific. Some individuals distinguish between "hard/natural sciences" (e.g., physics, chemistry, biology, astronomy, earth sciences) and "soft/social sciences" (e.g., psychology, sociology, anthropology, economics). The intersection between the sciences and the humanities (e.g., philosophy, history, literature, the arts) has historically played a role in these discussions. The term also is applied to fields that use scientific methods (e.g., nursing science, computer science, library science, environmental science).

Most simply, science may be thought of as an activity that combines research (the advancement of knowledge) and theory (the explanation for knowledge). A common way of compartmentalization is basic science versus applied science. The term *basic science* refers to the study of phenomena from a purely epistemological standpoint, regardless of any particular applications the findings might happen to have. *Applied science,* as the term implies, is oriented toward the solution of practical problems. The distinction is easiest to see in mathematics (where some very important theorems have absolutely no real-world representations) and in biology (where studies involving animals are called basic and studies involving humans are called applied).

Although science = research + theory, not all scientists are both researchers and theorists. It is fairly common practice in many sciences for a relatively small number of scientists to do most or all of the theorizing and for the others to carry out research that either generates or tests such theories. For example, although some theories used in nursing are *'borrowed' from or 'shared' with other disciplines, there *are* nursing theories, and there have been many research investigations that have generated such theories and/or subjected them to empirical testing.

See **Human Science, Research,** and **Theory.**

Secondary Analysis

Secondary analysis involves the creation of a research project based on a reanalysis of data previously collected for other purposes. There are a number of ways in which this research approach can be used effectively to produce new and important information. Research projects tend to yield more data than can be analyzed at one time. In addition to studying unanalyzed variables, the secondary investigator can test other aspects of relationships among variables or can examine particular subsamples. Data may also be organized differently for analysis. For example, the unit of analysis may be changed from distinct sets of individual responses to the aggregate, with individual responses merged and treated as a single unit, or vice versa. In addition, smaller or larger categories of data may be created that more closely relate to the current research interest or new hypothesis to be tested. The limitations of this approach involve those typically associated with use of existing data; that is, the secondary investigator has no control over how the data were collected, and in content, the data may not exactly suit the purposes of the proposed research.

Increasing use of computer technology has given rise to data banks that store survey data (although secondary analysis may also involve use of data collected by other means). Lists of data banks, which include both government and private sources, are obtainable. In the case of large-scale data sets, secondary analysis not only helps to extend the research potential of the original data but is also cost-effective.

In the case of smaller data sets, researchers sometimes indicate a willingness to make study data available to other investigators for the purpose of secondary analysis.

Kiecolt and Nathan (1985) have written an entire monograph devoted to secondary analysis of survey data. For examples of secondary analysis in nursing research see DiNapoli (2003) and Tang (2003).

Secondary Source

A *secondary source* is a source of data that consists of summarization of or commentary about primary data, such as writings or a life experience, by someone other than the person who produced the data or lived through the experience.

See **Primary Source.**

Semantic Differential

The *semantic differential* is a measurement strategy first introduced by Osgood, Suci, and Tannenbaum (1957) for assessing the connotative and denotative meanings of various concepts. The subject is given a number of concepts, such as love, ideal patient, and so forth and asked to rate

S

each concept on each of a number of bipolar scales, such as good/bad, strong/weak, and so forth. The purpose is to determine the distances between pairs of concepts in the 'semantic space' formed by those scales. Those concepts that are close together in that space are things that are perceived as similar in meaning and those that are far apart are things that have very little in common with one another.

The study by Bowles (1986) is a good example of the use of the semantic differential in nursing research.

Semiotics

Semiotics (also called semiology) is the study of signs, or more generally, the study of patterned communication systems. It represents 'the linguistic turn' in the philosophy of science, based on the seminal work of de Saussure (1857–1913), and is associated with structuralism and post-structuralism. All sorts of things (words, gestures, thoughts, sounds) can be 'signs' or 'signifiers' (i.e., symbols) that may be used to stand for something else. Pop culture (e.g., clothing and hairstyles, greeting cards, photography, film), forms of mass communication (e.g., television, radio), technologies, professional subcultures, and client communication (e.g., the way patients communicate symptoms and experiences) may be subjected to semiotic interpretation. A deconstructive poststructural interpretation involves stripping away layers of 'text' (meanings linked to signifiers) to expose the underlying premises and covert communications that call overt messages and themes into question. For classic works see Barthes (1984, 1986), Hawkes (1977), and Hebdige (1979). For use of the concept in nursing see Sandelowski (1999).

See **Deconstruction, Poststructuralism,** and **Structuralism.**

Sensitivity

The term *sensitivity* has at least three different, though weakly related, meanings in nursing research. Polit and Beck (2004) use the term in a *measurement* context. An instrument is said to be sensitive if it is capable of picking up fine distinctions in the measurement of a particular construct, for example, obesity. (A 'test' of obesity that can only categorize people as 'fat' or 'skinny' is not very sensitive.)

In addition to this use of the term as a property of a measuring instrument, there are two *statistical* contexts in which the notion of sensitivity arises. The first of these is in hypothesis testing, where a particular statistical analysis is called sensitive because, if the null hypothesis is false, the use of that analysis gives the researcher a high probability of arriving at the decision to reject it.

The second (and more common) statistical context in which the term *sensitivity* appears is in the analysis of data for certain kinds of epidemi-

S

ological research involving diagnostic testing. A distinction is made between the sensitivity of a diagnostic test (e.g., computerized tomography for detecting lung cancer) and the specificity of that test. Sensitivity is the proportion of a diseased group that the test successfully detects, and specificity is the proportion of a healthy group that the test successfully identifies as healthy. These definitions are equivalent to two terms used in statistical hypothesis-testing—the probability of *not* making a Type II error (often called the *power* of a test of statistical significance) and the probability of *not* making a Type I error. The terms *true positives* and *true negatives* are occasionally used in conjunction with *sensitivity* and *specificity*, respectively, although the complementary terms *false positives* (Type I errors) and *false negatives* (Type II errors) are more frequently encountered in the literature.

Example (of this third meaning of the term *sensitivity*): A diagnostic test for AIDS that has a sensitivity of .99 is very good indeed for determining that a person who actually has AIDS is correctly identified as having the disease. Unfortunately, however, the higher the sensitivity the lower the specificity (all other things being equal), so such a test might also identify as having AIDS a fairly sizable fraction of people who do not have the disease.

Sequential Analysis

Sequential analysis is an approach to statistical inference in which a variable (rather than fixed) sample size provides the basis for inferences that are made as the data accumulate. In sequential hypothesis-testing three (rather than two) decisions are made at each stage of data analysis with respect to the null hypothesis under investigation: accept it, reject it, or keep sampling.

Sequential analysis is particularly appropriate for clinical nursing research where subjects are entered into the study one at a time, subjects are in short supply, and measurements are expensive. It has been shown that on average the sample size required to test a particular effect is smaller for sequential analysis than for traditional forms of statistical inference.

For a comprehensive article that describes sequential hypothesis-testing, see Brown, Porter, and Knapp (1993).

Simultaneous Regression Analysis

Simultaneous regression analysis is a type of regression analysis in which all of the independent variables are 'entered' into the analysis at the same time.

Zachariah (1994) used simultaneous regression analysis in a study of maternal-fetal attachment.

See **Regression Analysis.**

Snowball Sampling

Snowball sampling is a type of nonprobability sampling in which subjects initially selected recruit other subjects, who in turn recruit still other subjects, and so forth.

For an example of the use of snowball sampling in nursing research, see Hitchcock and Wilson (1992).

See **Sampling.**

Specificity

In epidemiological research *specificity* is a term used to define the proportion of subjects correctly identified by some diagnostic procedure as not having a particular disease.

See **Sensitivity.**

Split Halves

Split halves is a method for assessing the internal consistency reliability of a set of test items. The researcher administers the test only once, but for scoring purposes, splits the test into two halves (ideally randomly, but usually by odd-numbered and even-numbered test questions) and obtains a score for each subject on each half. The scores on one half are then correlated with the scores on the other half, and the Spearman-Brown formula is applied to that correlation, yielding an estimate of the test's reliability. This technique is closely associated with Cronbach's coefficient alpha (which is the average of all possible split-half reliabilities) but is used less often in nursing research than alpha.

See **Reliability.**

Spurious Relationship

A *spurious relationship* is a relationship between two variables that vanishes when a third variable is taken into account.

Example: There is a very high positive correlation between height and reading ability of elementary school children. However, when age is taken into account (e.g., by the technique of partial correlation), that relationship is reduced very close to zero, because it is age that is 'driving' both variables.

Stakeholders

In some types of investigation, people recruited into the study are not considered to be 'subjects.' Rather, because they are seen as partners in the research process, they are called respondents, participants, or stakeholders. The term *stakeholder* is common to emancipatory forms of inquiry, such as feminist research. Here it implies an open, nonexploitive

S

researcher-participant relationship characterized by equality and mutuality. *Stakeholders* in evaluation research are groups and individuals who may be affected by and/or who have vested interests in or concerns about the program/practice under review.

See **Evaluation Research, Feminist Research,** and **Participatory Action Research.**

Standard Deviation

The *standard deviation* of a set of data for a variable is a descriptive statistic that summarizes the amount of variability around the mean. It is calculated by finding the mean of the squared deviations (differences) from the mean and then taking the square root. (The quantity obtained before taking the square root is called the variance. The standard deviation is the square root of the variance.) It can take on values from 0 (no variability at all) to one half of the range (maximum variability). It should always be reported whenever the mean is reported, because two frequency distributions could have the same mean but quite different standard deviations and therefore indicate different amounts of variability with respect to that mean.

Some authors of statistics textbooks define the standard deviation in a slightly different way. They divide by one less than the number of 'scores,' rather than the actual number of 'scores,' before extracting the square root. The reasons for this are very complicated; see, for example, Munro, 2001.

See **Range** and **Variance.**

Statistic

A *statistic* is a descriptive index for a sample, such as a sample mean, sample standard deviation, or sample correlation coefficient. It is contrasted with a parameter, which is the corresponding descriptive index for the entire population.

See **Parameter** and **Sample.**

Stepwise Regression Analysis

Stepwise regression analysis is a type of regression analysis that is different from, but often confused with, hierarchical regression analysis.

In stepwise regression analysis the independent variables are "entered" sequentially not according to any theory but strictly on the basis of statistical significance.

Ulrich, Soeken, and Miller (2003) used stepwise regression analysis in their study of ethical conflict and managed care.

See **Regression Analysis.**

Stratified Random Sampling

Stratified random sampling is a type of random sampling in which the population is divided into subpopulations or 'strata' on the basis of one or more variables and a simple random sample is drawn from each 'stratum.'

See **Sampling.**

Structural Equation Modeling (SEM)

Structural equation modeling (SEM) is an extension of path analysis to the situation in which both measured variables (sometimes called 'manifest' variables) and unmeasured variables (the underlying 'latent' variables, or factors) are of interest. The model has two parts: (a) the measurement model, in which the relationships between the manifest variables and their underlying latent counterparts are assessed; and (b) the structural model, in which the relationships between the latent variables are of prime concern.

The computer packages LISREL and EQS are usually employed to study both parts of the model. Pedhazur (1997) is a good source for understanding the basic concepts of structural equation modeling.

The application of the theory of planned behavior to the breastfeeding duration of Hong Kong mothers, carried out by Dodgson, Henly, Duckett, and Tarrant (2003), is a good example of the use of SEM.

Structural-Functionalism

See **Functionalism.**

Structuralism

Structuralism is best described as an intellectual movement, including scholars from many fields (e.g., linguistics, literary criticism, anthropology, sociology), which came to prominence in the 1950s–1960s, in part through the efforts of anthropologist Claude Levi-Strauss. It built on the work of linguist Ferdinand de Saussure (1857–1913) who, in his study of the underlying elements (the structure) of language, developed a system of sign analysis that he called *semiology (semiotics)*. Semiology was a starting point for structuralism and poststructuralism. In philosophy, this emphasis on language in cultural studies is called 'the linguistic turn.' Levi-Strauss adapted a style of linguistic analysis to the study of culture, proposing that many patterns underlying objects of culture, such as myths, marriage and kinship customs, rites, and relationships are elaborations of basic structures of the mind. Therefore, the focus on the individual was replaced by a focus on these structures believed to underlie the universal organization of human culture. (Objects of structural analysis varied by discipline—e.g., economic, psychological, historical—the above being only one example among many versions of structuralism.)

S

Structuralism was criticized for being *reductionistic (attempting to account for diversity and complexity by means of a single determining factor), static (preoccupied with abstract formal models), ahistorical (operating in the present), and anti-humanistic (unheeding of the feelings, actions, and intentions of individuals). It was eventually rejected in the 1980s by deconstruction and poststructuralism, which had been evolving contemporaneously with and in response to the tenets of structuralism.

See **Deconstruction, Poststructuralism,** and **Semiotics.**

Subject

In social research, *subject* has a very special meaning, to wit, the person who is being studied. (If there is more than one person, they are called, naturally enough, subjects.) The abbreviations S (for subject) and Ss (for subjects) are very commonly used, particularly in the psychological literature, along with E and Es for experimenter(s).

Animals used in basic research are occasionally also called subjects, but if inanimate things (hospital, county, etc.) are the units of analysis some other term is usually employed. A term sometimes used interchangeably with subject is *object,* which is indeed strange as the two words have quite different meanings in English grammar (subject-predicate-object) and in common parlance (e.g., a school subject such as history or the object of someone's affection).

Some people find the term *subject* a bit demeaning (conveying the impression that the person[s] being studied should be regarded as subservient to the researcher) and suggest the less pejorative term *participant.* Participants who in some types of research are viewed as partners and co-investigators are sometimes referred to as *stakeholders.

Universities in which scientific research is carried out have *Institutional Review Boards whose responsibility is to oversee the protection of the rights of study participants through such mechanisms as *informed consent, *anonymity, *confidentiality, and freedom to withdraw from the study without retaliation. However,

> [i]nvestigators bear the ultimate ethical responsibility for their work with human subjects. . . . Compliance with human subject protection regulations should not be seen as something that must be done just because it is required by the regulations. Compliance should be seen as the 'right thing to do' because it helps protect the rights and welfare of the subjects of human research and maintains public trust in research (Dunn & Chadwick, 2002, p. 26).

Subjective/Subjectivity

The term *subjective* refers to individual points of view and also is used, in a negative sense, to refer to 'bias' as undue prejudice for or against something. But, it does not follow that 'bias' is inherently negative. Rather, it is the explicit recognition that one has a point of view. Contradictions call to mind how, in the history of scientific inquiry, the classic opposition has been characterized as being between *objectivity* (the goal of science, free of bias and prejudice) and *subjectivity* (the threat of prejudicial feelings and biased impressions). However, there has been increasing appreciation for how the subjectivity of research subjects' accounts informs investigations and how the researcher's subjectivity (i.e., reflexive awareness and use of self) brings this understanding forward. Indeed, postmodern thinking is less in favor of retaining ideas about the *subject/object dualism* and more in favor of the perspective that our knowledge of the world, ourselves, and others is neither *subjective nor objective,* but both in a form of reflexive-dialectical interaction as inseparable and mutually supportive aspects of the same reality.

See **Objective/Objectivity** and **Subjectivism.**

Subjectivism

Subjectivism is the epistemological view that reality is not independent of human perception and belief. Therefore (in contrast to objectivism), because inquiry cannot avoid being influenced by the investigator's values, it must be in the form of a dialogue. *Interpretivism and constructivism are two examples of philosophies that assume a subjectivist epistemology. However, there are many different subjectivist epistemological stances, some of which are related and others of which are at odds with one another over a wide variety of philosophical and methodological issues.

See **Constructivism/Constructionalism, Epistemology,** and **Objectivism.**

Substantive Theory

A *substantive theory* is at a level that is close to a specific problem and/or population. Many *ethnographic and *grounded theory studies, for example, generate substantive theories that provide "rich, meaningful . . . theoretical models of individuals' perspectives on a given phenomenon and the process or strategies they use to resolve or cope with the problem in a distinct and bounded context" (Kearney, 1998, p. 179). *Substantive theory* is "a strategic link in the formulation and development of *formal theory* based on data" (Glaser & Strauss, 1967, p. 34).

See **Formal Theory.**

Survey

The term *survey* has two equally common meanings. Half of the scientific community defines a survey as research that involves questionnaires and/or interviews and large numbers of respondents. The other half of the scientific community defines a survey as any research based on a probability sample, that is, a sample drawn from a population in such a way that every object has a known probability of being selected.

For those who adopt the latter definition, the survey may or may not involve questionnaires or interviews, and may or may not involve large numbers of participants. For example, a study in which a simple random sample of 112 adult males are weighed would be regarded by this 'camp' as survey research, whereas the questionnaire/interview 'camp' would call that sort of study something else ('descriptive research' is a popular catchall category).

Surveys that involve a series of questions in interview or questionnaire format are usually conducted for the general purpose of obtaining information about practices, opinions, attitudes, and other characteristics of people. Survey researchers typically collect a broad range of demographic data on participants' backgrounds as well. Although these data may not be central to the study, they may help to explain the study findings, because background characteristics frequently can be linked with behavioral and attitudinal patterns. The most basic function of a survey is description, although explanation of why people behave or believe as they do and prediction of responses with regard to the variable(s) of interest may be additional objectives.

A number of designs may be used in surveys. The main concerns are with sampling procedures, sample size, and instrument validity and reliability. Researchers try to obtain as large a sample as necessary to minimize sampling error and to allow for a certain percentage of nonresponse. Careful construction of interview schedules and questionnaires, and pilot testing of these instruments, is essential. A pilot study based on a small preliminary sample can alert the researcher to questions that may need to be changed or deleted, additional questions that should be included, or other logistical revisions.

An advantage of surveys is that large amounts of data can be amassed. A disadvantage is that the actual information content can be fairly superficial. The researcher must determine if study interests are best served by an extensive survey focused on selected variables or by an intensive examination (case study) of more variables with a small sample or single subject. Because the investigator usually has little control over the research situation, causal relationships are more difficult to establish in surveys than in true experiments. However, carefully designed surveys are almost always objective, are a good source of hypotheses, and can suggest directions for further research.

Example (of a study that would satisfy both definitions): A researcher interested in the smoking behavior of nurses might draw a probability sample of 1,000 nurses listed in the latest edition of the American Nurses

S

Association (ANA) directory and send out a questionnaire to each of those nurses asking for information regarding whether or not they smoke cigarettes, how many they smoke, and so forth.

Bliss, Fischer, Savik, Avery, and Mark (2004) reported the results of an anonymous survey concerning the severity of fecal incontinence.

Survival Analysis

Survival analysis is a complicated statistical analysis applied to certain epidemiological studies in which the "endpoint" (survival, death, etc.) has not yet been reached for all of the subjects who participated in the study. For such subjects it is unclear whether and/or when the endpoint will occur.

Koniak-Griffin, Verzemnieks, Anderson, Brecht, Lesser, Kim, et al. (2003) used survival analysis in their two-year study of nurse visitations to adolescent mothers.

Symbolic Interaction

Symbolic interaction is a theoretical perspective associated with the "Chicago school," that is, the University of Chicago Department of Sociology and scholarly work emanating from it for over 20 years between World War I and the mid-1930s. During this period the Chicago school dominated American sociology. Symbolic interaction was one of the many emphases in Chicago sociology at this time. It originated with pragmatist philosopher and social psychologist George Herbert Mead (1863–1931). From 1894 until his death in 1931, Mead taught courses in the philosophy department at Chicago that were attended by many graduate students in sociology. His ideas so profoundly affected them that they put together their lecture notes and published a posthumous volume under his name. Symbolic interaction (SI) was created from this effort. Herbert Blumer coined the phrase and advocated SI in the Meadian tradition at Chicago in the 1940s and 1950s.

Symbolic interaction provided an alternative to the dominance of functionalism and social systems theory with their emphasis on equilibrium models. These latter perspectives focused on explaining social behavior according to the role or function it served in the larger society but neglected to account for individual motives and the meanings people give to their actions. In Mead's philosophy, a person's sense of self emerges through social interaction. The relationship between self and society is an ongoing process of symbolic communication. A sense of self develops as people (a) imagine themselves in other social roles (seeing themselves through others' eyes and internalizing the attitudes of the generalized other), (b) anticipate the responses of others, and (c) act in accordance with the meaning that things (other people, ideas, events, objects, or situations) have for them. Thus, through thought and action, people are continuously creating social reality. But they are rarely aware of these ordinary processes embedded in the natural flow of everyday life.

Symbolic interactionists advocated methods that would allow researchers to explore the meanings hidden in the social world of the individual. Grounded theory method, developed by Glaser and Strauss (1967), takes a symbolic interactionist perspective. The Chicago school ethnographic studies of urban life also were linked with it in their concern with identity formation, which was thought to be the result of people's self-perceptions in combination with how they thought others viewed them. And Erving Goffman (1922–1982), a student of Blumer at Chicago, developed dramaturgical analysis as a variation of symbolic interaction, where interpretation of social behavior takes a view of life as theater. The assumption is that when people interact, they want to manage others' impressions of themselves. Consequently, they give performances, enact parts or routines, make use of environment for setting and props, and control what is stage front and backstage (hidden from the audience). The central concern in Goffman's work is the self in society. The drama of everyday life lies in its fragility and its potential for disruption by misunderstandings, embarrassments, uncertainties, and similar tensions that routinely occur in face-to-face encounters of varying duration. Systems and people in systems are constantly working to maintain mechanisms that prevent tensions from becoming too severe and overwhelming the balance needed to sustain social interaction.

The symbolic focus on role and communication has influenced studies of the sociology of illness behavior, patient-care provider interaction, and the role of social factors in health care systems. For additional background see Blumer (1969), Glaser and Strauss (1967), Goffman (1959, 1967), and Mead (1934, 1938, 1959).

See **Grounded Theory** and **Pragmatism.**

Systematic Reviews

Systematic reviews are overviews of research evidence that address a specific clinical question and use

> a detailed, comprehensive search strategy and rigorous appraisal methods for the purpose of summarizing, appraising, and communicating the results and implications of contradictory results or otherwise unmanageable quantities of research. . . . Systematic reviews of RCTs [randomized clinical trials], considered Level I evidence, are found at the top of the hierarchy of evidence (Melnyk, 2003) (Johnston, 2005, p. 115).

Meta-analyses and *metasyntheses* are types of systematic reviews. An *integrative review* also is a systematic review "that does not have a summary statistic because sample sizes cannot be summarized in an integrative review (usually due to heterogeneous studies/samples [e.g., experimental, theory, and descriptive studies]" (Johnston, p. 115). However, systematic reviews are not the same as *literature reviews* that are done for the purpose of providing background information on an issue. See Johnston (2005) for a more detailed discussion of the process of undertaking a systematic review; McInnes and Askie (2004) for an example of a systematic review of qualitative and quantitative reviews that focus on older people's views and experiences of falls prevention; Elliott, Staniunas, Rajab, Marcus, and Snyder (2004) for a review of systematic reviews on the effectiveness of public health nursing; Fager and Melnyk (2004) for an integrative review of intervention studies targeted at decreasing alcohol use in college students; and Chiu, Emblen, Hofwegen, Sawatzky, and Meyerhoff (2004) for an integrative review of how the concept of spirituality has been reported in the health sciences literature in the past decade.

Systematic Sampling

Systematic sampling is a type of sampling in which every kth (where k is some convenient number) member of the population is selected into the sample.

Floyd (1993) has written a very comprehensive article on systematic sampling. See also Levy and Lemeshow (1999).

See **Sampling.**

S

T

t test

The *t test* is a very popular test of statistical significance for assessing the difference between two sample means. The samples are usually independent, but occasionally they are dependent (correlated, matched, paired).

Janke (1994) used a *t* test (one-tailed) in one of the analyses she carried out regarding the development of an instrument for predicting breast-feeding attrition.

See Test of Significance.

Test of Significance

A *test of significance* is a statistical hypothesis-testing procedure for determining the extent to which a particular sample result may be attributable to chance.

Such a test involves the postulation of a null (chance) hypothesis (e.g., that there is no relationship between X and Y) and an alternative hypothesis (usually arising from some sort of theory) regarding the population of interest. A sample is drawn from the population, a statistic is calculated for that sample, and a decision is made to reject or not to reject the null hypothesis. If the null hypothesis is rejected, the sample result is said to be statistically significant.

If a true null hypothesis is rejected (the researcher never knows whether it is true or false, but must entertain both possibilities), a Type I error is said to have been made. If a false null hypothesis is not rejected, a Type II error is said to have been made. The probabilities of making these kinds of errors are called alpha errors (Type I) and beta errors (Type II) because of the Greek symbols used to denote them. The probability of making a Type I error is also called the level of significance. The complement of the probability of making a Type II error, that is, 1 − beta, is called the power of the test of significance.

The researcher usually tries to keep both alpha and beta small (conventionally around .05 or so), but unfortunately as one decreases the other increases, all other things being equal. The only way to minimize both of them is to draw a very large sample size (take a bigger 'chunk' out of the population). That can be expensive and often leads to statistically significant but not very important results.

If the alternative hypothesis is 'directional' or 'one-sided' (e.g., there is an inverse relationship between X and Y), a 'one-tailed test' is called for. If the alternative hypothesis is nondirectional (e.g., there is a relationship between X and Y), a 'two-tailed test' is called for. Those names derive from the area of the sampling distribution in which the 'rejection region' (alpha region) for the test is located.

The most commonly encountered tests of significance are the t test for the difference between two sample means, the analysis of variance F test for several sample means, the analysis of covariance F test for 'adjusted' sample means, and the chi-square test of the relationship between two nominal variables.

All four of those procedures involve the concept of 'degrees of freedom' (df), a term associated with the corresponding sampling distributions (t, F, or chi-square) that are used to carry out the tests.

Example: If the null hypothesis of no relationship between age and pulse rate were tested against the alternative hypothesis of an inverse relationship between the two, and a sample of 1,000 observations yielded a correlation coefficient of –.08, the null hypothesis would be rejected in favor of the alternative, and the result would be statistically significant at the .01 level, but the finding would undoubtedly not be regarded as very important because the sample correlation is so close to zero.

Test-Retest

Test-retest is a procedure for assessing the reliability (stability) of a measuring instrument.

See **Reliability.**

Theorem

In mathematics and logic, a *theorem* is a conclusion, drawn from a set of axioms within a logical deductive framework, which is accepted as truth. Theorems and axioms are considered to be less tentative than other types of propositional statements.

See **Theory, Axiom,** and **Proposition.**

Theoretical Perspective

A *theoretical perspective* is an orienting philosophical framework that, in scientific inquiry, is informed by epistemology (a theory of knowledge) and, in turn, guides researchers' chosen research methodologies. It is one of four interrelated research elements discussed by Crotty (1998, pp. 2–5, 7–8). Out of many theoretical stances, he gives as examples positivism/postpositivism, interpretivism (symbolic interaction, phenomenology, hermeneutics), critical inquiry, feminism, and postmodernism.

See **Research.**

Theoretical Sampling

Theoretical sampling is a type of purposeful sampling that is used in *grounded theory research. As data are concurrently collected and analyzed, the researcher decides what further information is needed to develop the emerging theory. Charmaz (2000) observes: "Although we often sample people, we may sample scenes, events, or documents, depending on the study and where the theory leads us" (p. 519). See Norton and Bowers's (2001) research on end-of-life decision making for a sense of the interplay between theoretical sampling and theory development.

See **Purposeful Sampling.**

Theory

Elements of theory: A *theory* is a set of statements that tentatively describe, explain, or predict relationships between concepts that have been systematically selected and organized as an abstract representation of some phenomenon. *Concepts, sometimes called the *building blocks of theory,* are the major ideas expressed by the theory. Concept development and testing of theoretical relationships through research involve defining concepts in relation to their *empirical indicators or referents (those properties of concepts that can be verified). The means to accomplish this may be fairly direct in the case of concrete concepts (e.g., sex, weight, height); but abstract concepts (e.g., hope, anxiety, self-esteem) will involve more indirect measures and multiple empirical indicators. For example, Polit and Beck (2004, p. 32) describe different empirical indicators that researchers might choose to measure *anxiety* depending on what aspects of this concept they wish to emphasize (e.g., Palmar Sweat Index as a physiological measure; State Anxiety Scale as a measure of psychological state).

*Propositions are statements about the relationships between two or more concepts. In the logical development of theories, it is expected that propositions will follow a clearly identifiable line of reasoning from initial premises to conclusions. Some specific types of propositions are *postulates, *premises, and *axioms, which in a formal logical deductive format are introductory propositional statements. Axioms as premises are presumed to be true, in contrast to the tentative nature of most propositions. Other types of propositions are *theorems, *hypotheses, and *laws, which in a chain of logical deductive reasoning are <u>concluding propositional statements</u>. Theorems are derived from axioms and more usually pertain to the science of mathematics. Because axioms as premises connote a greater degree of certainty, theorems also will be considered as less tentative than hypotheses. Hypotheses are propositional statements that are tested by means of systematic research approaches. Supported hypotheses may also serve as premises in deductive arguments, where they lend a higher degree of soundness to conclusions than do untested premises. Patterns of relationships that have become widely accepted by virtue of repeated validation through research may be called laws. A law is a propositional statement that is highly generalizable, that is, consistently supported and therefore not tentative (Chinn & Kramer, 1995, p. 216). In comparison to the physical sciences, the social/human sciences have relatively few laws.

<u>The nature of theory</u>: It is important to appreciate the tentative nature of theory. Theory is not reality; it is an abstraction of reality based on assumptions about the true nature of a phenomenon that cannot be proved or disproved. The degree of support that may be found for a theory relies on applying various forms of reasoning to test the logic of propositional statements and validating associated hypotheses through research.

<u>Theory and research</u>: Theory-linked research is designed to generate, test/validate, or refine theory (Chinn & Kramer, 2004). Theory-generating research tends to be qualitative in design (e.g., grounded theory or ethnographic field research) and, initially, inductive in nature. Theory-testing/validating research tends to be quantitative in design (e.g., descriptive, correlational, hypothesis-testing), and primarily, deductive in nature. Research designed specifically to refine concepts and theoretic relationships (i.e., validating empiric indicators for theory concepts, empirically grounding emerging relationships, and empirically validating relationships) involves both qualitative and quantitative approaches (Chinn & Kramer). "These types of investigations are crucial early in the stages of a theory's development but can be used at any point of theoretic development" (p. 125).

<u>Common nursing themes</u>: Original theoretical thinking, apart from processes of research, is a source of many theories in the social and human sciences. In nursing, theoretical thinking about the discipline's nature, mission, and goals can be found in the writings of Nightingale and an ongoing legacy of 'nurse theorists' whose earliest work was directed toward mapping the discipline's domain, that is, defining its practice concerns and developing teaching strategies. Thus, conceptualizations of nursing as a profession have addressed frequently recurring and common themes. Yura and Torres (1975) and Fawcett (1984) identified common

themes in terms of four concepts that constitute the *metaparadigm (domain) of nursing (person, environment, health, and nursing). More recently, Fawcett (2000) has defined each concept and formalized the themes into propositions which, taken together, constitute the mission and substance of nursing.

Nurse theorists: Nursing *models and theories provide many different ways of looking at the phenomena of interest to the discipline. Historically best-known nursing conceptual models and theories include: Nightingale's notes on nursing; Peplau's interpersonal relations model; Henderson's principles and practice of nursing; Johnson's behavioral system model; Orem's self-care framework and self-care deficit nursing theory; Abdellah's patient-centered approaches to nursing; Hall's care, core, and cure model; Paterson and Zderad's humanistic nursing theory; Orlando's (Pelletier's) theory of the dynamic nurse-patient relationship/deliberative nursing process; Travelbee's nurse-patient relationship; Wiedenbach's theory of nursing as a helping art; Levine's conservation model; King's general systems framework and theory of goal attainment; Rogers's science of unitary man; Roy's adaptation model; Riehl's interaction model; Neuman's systems model; Parse's human becoming theory; Newman's theory of health as expanding consciousness; Watson's theory of human caring; Leininger's theory of culture care diversity; and Benner and Wrubel's primacy of caring in nursing (Chinn & Kramer, 2004; Fawcett, 2000; Fitzpatrick & Whall, 1996; Hinton Walker & Neuman, 1996; McEwen & Wills, 2002; Meleis, 1997; Parker, M., 2001).

Evaluation and classification: Nursing models and theories have been analyzed and evaluated in terms of their paradigmatic origins (historical evolution and worldviews); underlying assumptions; scope (complexity and degree of abstraction); major concepts and primary focus; underlying structure (clarity, consistency, and logical development of major elements: context, content, process, and goals); social significance and practical utility; contrasting and competing views; and fit or blueprint for implementation in research, education, practice, and administration settings and projects (Barnum, 1998; Fawcett, 2000; Hinton Walker & Neuman, 1996; McEwen & Wills, 2002; Meleis, 1997). They also have been classified along a variety of different dimensions. For example, a focus on images of nursing in sociocultural context is illustrated by Meleis' (1997) groupings of theorists by *schools of thought* (1950–1970)—the "needs theorists" (Abdellah, Henderson, Orem) who described nursing as meeting the needs of clients, the "interaction theorists" (King, Orlando, Paterson and Zderad, Peplau, Travelbee, and Wiedenbach) who saw nursing as supporting and promoting interactions with patients, and the "outcome theorists" (Johnson, Levine, Rogers, Roy) who focused on the end result of caring processes and then described the recipient of

T

the care (Meleis, 1997, pp. 185–195). In contrast, scope and level of development served Fawcett's (2000) need to differentiate conceptual models of nursing (Johnson, King, Levine, Neuman, Orem, Rogers, Roy), grand nursing theories (Leininger, Newman, Parse), and middle-range nursing theories (Orlando, Peplau, Watson). Thus, classifications of nursing theories involve choices that serve different purposes; and some authors do not intend them to be mutually exclusive or inclusive.

<u>Primary sources</u>: There are many general texts that do an excellent job of interpreting theory development in nursing in historical perspective, while providing guidance in analyzing, and evaluating individual theories. However, it is preferable to read theorists' original works rather than to rely solely on others' interpretations of them.

<u>Issues and applications</u>: In addition to comprehensive surveys and analyses of extant theories of varying types, there are works such as Barnum's (1998), that analyzes what has been written about theory (*metatheory) and uses multiple theory works to sensitize readers to the theoretical implications of common nursing practice concerns (e.g., traditions in caring, spirituality and ethics in nursing). Other texts emphasize application of theory such as McEwen and Wills's (2002) work that offers an overview of grand (*broad-range) theories in nursing while addressing in detail the concrete application of *middle-range and practice-oriented theories. Similarly, Smith and Liehr (2003) discuss applications of eight middle-range nursing theories, and Fawcett (2000) introduces the idea of a comprehensive conceptual-theoretical-empirical system (C-T-E system) of nursing knowledge as a strategy to promote the integration of theory, practice, and research for the future of the discipline.

<u>Theory/knowledge development</u>: Another segment of the theory literature is concerned with theory development. For example, H. S. Kim (2000) provides a typology (four conceptual fields) to be used as a mapping device for theorizing about phenomena of interest to nursing. Walker and Avant's (2005) three-stage strategies for theory construction in nursing offer a procedural focus on development of three basic elements of theory building, that is, *concept, statement,* and *theory* through processes of (a) synthesis, (b) derivation, and (c) analysis. Rodgers and Knafl (2000) focus on techniques and applications of *concept development. And, Chinn and Kramer (2004) address *Integrated Knowledge Development in Nursing* based on the four fundamental *patterns of knowing described by Carper (1978) as critical components of the discipline, that is, empirical knowing (the science of nursing), ethical knowing (the moral component in nursing), personal knowing (knowing self/others), and aesthetic knowing (the art of nursing).

Thick Description

The concept of *thick description* often is invoked as a criterion for good ethnographic writing. However, it is not (as some suppose) a synonym for rich, detailed description. Rather, it refers to an analytic stance that is specific to cultural interpretation. Geertz (1973) emphasized that

> this . . . is not a matter of methods [techniques] . . . What defines [an ethnographic interpretation] is the kind of intellectual effort it is: an elaborate venture in, to borrow a notion from Gilbert Ryle, *thick description* . . . [That is] sorting out the structures of signification . . . established codes [inherent in human situations] and determining their social ground and import (pp. 6, 9).

Thick (as opposed to *thin*) description is rich in expression and detail; but the description is part of the process and always in service to a cultural interpretation of meaning in context.

See **Ethnography, Interpretation,** and **Contextualism.**

Transcription

A *transcription* is some kind of a written text. It may be an extended fieldnote. Often the term is associated with transcriptions of audiotaped material. Regardless of the skill and experience of the transcriptionist, transcripts need to be checked carefully for accuracy against the original recordings. Easton, McComish, and Greenberg (2000) describe how transcripts are prone to many common errors. MacLean, Meyer, and Estable (2004) offer suggestions for improving accuracy and discuss issues that include: the use of voice recognition systems; notation choices; the human factor; processing and active listening versus touch typing; transcriptionist effect; emotionally loaded audiotaped material; class and/or cultural differences among interviewee, interviewer, and transcriptionist; and errors that arise when working in a second language. For completeness, transcripts of audiotaped interviews should be accompanied by *fieldnotes that compensate for the fact that transcriptions are only partial accounts of the interaction, devoid of nonverbal elements and the researcher's observations and reflections.

See **Intensive (In-Depth) Interviewing.**

Transferability

See **Trustworthiness Criteria.**

Translational Research

Translational research involves the translation of basic research knowledge into clinical applications. Titler (2004) defines it as:

T

the scientific investigation of methods and variables that affect adoption of evidence-based health care practices by individual practitioners and health care systems to improve clinical and operational decision making . . . This includes testing the effect of interventions to promote and sustain adoption of evidence-based practices (EBPs) (p. 38).

This article reviews four *exemplars of translation studies and discusses research methods to advance knowledge about the efficacy of translating research into practice (TRIP) interventions.

Treatment Effects

The results of an experiment, especially for a clinical trial, are often referred to as *treatment effects,* that is, the effects of the various interventions relative to one another. The effects can range in magnitude from none to very strong.

See **Clinical Trial** and **Experiment.**

Triangulation

Triangulation is a term that is used in a number of fields, such as surveying, radio broadcasting, astronomy, and navigation, to describe a process of determining distance between various points by dividing up a large area into a series of connected triangles. In research, it refers to a variety of techniques used to ensure the *validity of data. Some alternative terms include multiple operationalism, operational delineation, convergent validation (in educational and psychological testing), corroboration, cross-validation, and multiple validation. Because the concept is used in many different ways, researchers need to be sure to specify its meaning and purpose in relation to their work and cite the literature that is consistent with that orientation.

In qualitative research, 'data' and 'methodological triangulation' (use of a variety of data sources and data gathering techniques) is a long-standing *fieldwork norm; but 'triangulation' has not been a traditional term for that. Discussions about 'triangulation' became fashionable in the 1980s and 1990s when types of triangulation that could be used in a single study were described as: (a) investigator triangulation (the use of researchers with different skill sets); (b) data triangulation (as defined above); (c) theory triangulation (use of multiple theoretical perspectives); and methodological triangulation (as defined above and also extended to later discussions about *mixed methods research). Many qualitative researchers are in agreement with Richardson (1994) "who offers the idea of crystallization as a better lens through which to view [multi-faceted] qualitative research designs and their components" (Janesick, 2000, p. 392). However, researchers continue to find the concept of

T

triangulation useful in their work. See, for instance, Kushner and Morrow's (2003) argument for linking grounded theory and feminist theory with critical theory (an example of *theoretical triangulation*). See also Shin, Pender, and Yun's (2003) use of *methodological triangulation* of qualitative and quantitative approaches as a research strategy for cultural verification of Pender's Planning for Exercise scale.

See **Mixed Methods Research.**

True Experiment

A *true experiment* is an experiment that is characterized by manipulation, random assignment, and other controls.

See **Experiment.**

True Score

A *true score* is a score that a subject 'deserves' to get on a test. It may differ from the score she or he actually obtains, however, due to the unreliability of the measuring instrument.

See **Reliability.**

Trustworthiness Criteria

Lincoln and Guba's (1985) following four *trustworthiness criteria* are the qualitative equivalents of concerns about *validity, *reliability, and *objectivity in quantitative research. (a) *Credibility* (paralleling internal validity) is demonstrated by <u>accuracy and validity</u> of findings that are assured through documentation of researcher actions, opinions, and biases; *<u>negative case analysis</u> (e.g., accounting for outliers/exceptions); <u>appropriateness</u> of data (e.g., *purposeful sampling, intensive engagement with and observation of the phenomenon); <u>adequacy of the database</u> (e.g., *saturation); <u>verification/corroboration</u> by use of multiple data sources (e.g., *triangulation); validation of data by informants (e.g., member checks); and <u>consultation</u> with colleagues (e.g., *peer debriefing). (b) *Transferability* (paralleling external validity) is demonstrated by a report that contains sufficient information for readers to determine whether findings are meaningful to other persons in similar situations (analytic or theoretical vs. statistical generalizability). (c) *Dependability* (paralleling reliability) is demonstrated by a research process that is carefully documented to provide evidence of how conclusions were reached and whether, under similar circumstances, another researcher might expect to obtain similar findings (i.e., the concept of the <u>audit trail</u>). (d) *Confirmability* (paralleling objectivity) is demonstrated by providing substantiation that findings and interpretations are grounded in the data (i.e., links between researcher assertions and the data are clear and

T

credible) and that the *audit trail is complete, comprehensible, useful, and linked to the methodological approach that was used (i.e., confirmation of *auditability*).

Although these analogs of quantitative evaluative criteria are widely used and cited, researchers may describe what they have done to ensure the rigor of their research without using the above terminology. They may clarify the procedures they have used in terms of *validity* and *reliability*; and they may apply *authenticity criteria,* which extend beyond purely methodological concerns. They also may prefer to use method-specific language, particularly in instances where the trustworthiness criteria do not apply as well (e.g., phenomenology, critical inquiry); and they will use common procedures and techniques recommended to enhance validity and *generalizability selectively. See, for example, Sandelowski's (1993, 1998) and Morse's (1998a) discussions about the problem with the use of *member checks and external reviewers to judge the validity of an interpretation. Morse, Barrett, Mayan, Olson, and Spiers (2002) further emphasize that methodological rigor is not a matter of 'post-hoc' evaluation at the end of the study. They argue that it is researcher 'responsiveness' to changing needs and potential problems while the study is ongoing that ensures the effectiveness of verification strategies (p. 5).

See **Authenticity Criteria** and **Validity.**

T

Two-Tailed Test

A *two-tailed test* is a test of statistical significance in which a null hypothesis is pitted against a nondirectional alternative hypothesis. A two-tailed test would be used if the alternative hypothesis to a null hypothesis of no relationship were simply that there is a relationship.

See **Alternative Hypothesis, Null Hypothesis,** and **Test of Significance.**

Type I Error

In a test of statistical significance a *Type I error* is defined as the rejection of a true null hypothesis.

See **Test of Significance.**

Type II Error

In a test of statistical significance a *Type II error* is defined as the nonrejection ('acceptance') of a false null hypothesis.

See **Test of Significance.**

U

Unit of Analysis

The term *unit of analysis* has at least two different meanings in research. The first and more common meaning is the 'thing' for which measurements have been obtained and subsequently subjected to data analysis. The unit might be a person (patient or nurse, for example), hospital, city, or virtually anything.

Occasionally the data may only be available for one unit of analysis, such as the hospital, but the researcher's interest may be in some other unit, such as the patient. Suppose that the research question is: "What is the relationship between amount of Demerol used and amount of reduction in pain?" For each of a number of *hospitals* we might know how much Demerol is dispensed each day and what percentage of the patients who take it each day actually experience pain reduction. But that is probably the wrong unit. We would like to know for each *patient* how much Demerol was used and whether or not she or he experienced any reduction in pain. If the *hospital* measurements are analyzed and the interpretation is made for the *patient,* a serious error could be committed, because the relationship could be quite different if the data were analyzed for individual patients. (Such an error is called an 'ecological fallacy.')

Some authors (e.g., Polit & Beck, 2004) use the term *unit of analysis* in a different sense. In content analysis the term is applied to the type of quantity being measured rather than the type of object on which the measurement is based.

Example: "What is the relationship between the heights and the weights of twins?" is a very difficult research question to answer because the unit of analysis could be an individual person or a pair of persons (if the latter, whose height and whose weight would be used?) and the two approaches could produce quite different results.

Unobtrusive Research

Unobtrusive research is research that is carried out on people who are unaware that they are being studied. It can take a variety of forms ranging from research involving hidden hardware (e.g., bedroom 'bugging' for the purpose of studying sexual behavior) to *archival research involving public records (e.g., birth certificates for studying the relationship between mother's age and baby's birth weight). More recently, the opportunity for unobtrusive internet-based research raises many ethical concerns. We have included a separate entry for *internet research*.

There is an entire book devoted to unobtrusive research (Webb, Campbell, Schwartz, Sechrest, & Grove, 1981). The principal advantages of such research are the lack of artificiality in what is studied and the inability of the subjects to refuse to cooperate in the research. The principal disadvantages are ethical ones (there are some serious moral and legal problems associated with bedroom bugging, for example), but for certain unobtrusive procedures there also are some sticky methodological problems. In a study of fascination with baby nurseries carried out by measuring smudges on the glass, you never know whether the smudges have been made by the same person spending a great deal of time watching the babies or by several persons all spending a short amount of time each. The same holds true if you want to use the wear and tear on library books as a measure of popularity. (There is also the additional problem, of course, that a particular book may be badly worn but never actually read!)

Some observational research is unobtrusive, but much is not. It is more common for researchers to obtain the explicit permission of the 'observees' than it is for them to carry out their observations without the knowledge of the subjects being studied. Field researchers are often *participant observers and as such they usually cannot make their observations unobtrusively.

As far as the advancement of knowledge regarding a particular phenomenon is concerned, a fruitful strategy might be to combine both obtrusive (e.g., interview) and unobtrusive (e.g., archival) approaches in order to get a double 'fix' on the problem. This strategy is a special case of *triangulation*.

Example: For many years people who took standardized multiple-choice tests were asked to blacken in the space between vertical dotted lines when recording their answers. More recently they have been asked to blacken in small ovals. Does it matter? A very nice unobtrusive (and perfectly ethical) controlled experiment could be carried out by randomly distributing answer sheets to a group of people being tested, with half of them getting the vertical dotted lines and the other half getting the ovals. Neither subgroup would know that everyone was not getting the same response form, much less that they were participating in an experiment, thereby avoiding the dreaded *Hawthorne Effect (see separate entry) that can often plague obtrusive research.

See **Internet Research.**

V

Validity

Validity is one of the two most important characteristics of a measuring instrument (the other is reliability). An instrument is said to be a *valid* way of operationalizing a construct if it really does measure that construct.

The literature is replete with procedures for determining whether or not, or to what extent, an instrument is valid, but they are all subsumed under three general types:

1. *Content validity* is concerned with the subjective determination of validity, usually by some sort of expert judgment, but alternatively or additionally by the persons being measured (the term face validity is used in the latter case).

2. In *criterion-related validity*, the measures obtained are compared with some external criterion that has itself already been judged to be valid (the "gold standard"). Some authors use the terms *concurrent validity* and *predictive validity* to distinguish between situations where the criterion data are gathered at about the same time as the measures for the instrument whose validity is in question and situations where the criterion data are gathered later.

3. *Construct validity* is concerned with theoretically based relationships that should pertain between measures produced by the instrument and measures of the same and other constructs.

Campbell and Fiske (1959) used the terms *convergent validity* and *discriminant validity* to refer to relationships with alleged measures of the same construct and relationships with alleged measures of other constructs, respectively.

The term *validity* is also used in the context of research design. An experimental study is said to be internally valid if the effect on the dependent variable can actually be attributed to the independent variable that has been manipulated, and not to some uncontrolled competing threat(s). Any study is said to be externally valid if the results are generalizable to persons and conditions other than those directly involved in the study.

In certain kinds of research there is the need for cross-validation of the findings. Regression analyses are particularly prone to 'overfitting' the sample data, so whenever possible one should divide the subjects randomly into two groups, derive the regression coefficients for each of the two groups separately, and then determine how well Group A's regression equation 'predicts' Group B's scores on the dependent variable, and vice versa.

Example: The 'mirror test' is one way of measuring obesity (look at yourself in a mirror and determine whether you're obese or not) and is generally regarded as content valid. The use of calipers to determine skin fold thickness is a more objective, but also content-valid, way of measuring obesity. It could serve as an external criterion for determining the criterion-related validity of indirect measures of obesity such as the body mass index (weight divided by the square of height). Also any instrument for measuring obesity should correlate positively with variables such as caloric intake and waist circumference, but should not correlate with variables such as body temperature if those instruments are to have acceptable construct validity.

Qualitative researchers often use other terms such as *truth value, credibility, trustworthiness,* and *accuracy* to describe their concerns about the soundness of their data (see entry for *trustworthiness criteria*). Ways of managing threats to 'internal validity' (the term is not used in the Campbell & Stanley, 1966, sense), for example, subject bias, reactive effect of the researcher, and changes in the study situation over time, are built into data collection and analysis procedures. These procedures include detailed record keeping, analytic notes accounting for the researcher's personal actions and subjective thoughts or impressions, multiple data sources, verification of data, and the simultaneous collection and analysis of data to examine their adequacy, to correct inaccuracies and imbalances, and assess transferability (paralleling external validity) of findings.

There are many different activities that qualitative researchers build into the designs of their studies to ensure that data are appropriate, adequate, and accurate. The selection of verification criteria is determined by the design and special needs of the study. Thus, the necessity for internal researcher-directed flexibility when referencing overall externally voiced standards should be recognized. However, Lincoln and Guba's (1985) *trustworthiness criteria,* followed by Guba and Lincoln's (1989) *authenticity criteria* are useful reference points. Later syntheses of crite-

V

ria commonly used to evaluate qualitative reports (e.g., Maxwell, 1992, and Whittemore, Chase, & Mandle, 2001) offer other ways to conceptualize what researchers do to assure quality and rigor. However, as efforts to be comprehensive intensify, conceptualizations and accompanying terminology expand and compete. Consequently, some researchers argue that developing alternative criteria in lieu of clarifying qualitative researchers' different approaches to *validity* (and *reliability*) does not adequately address issues pertaining to rigor and marginalizes the qualitative research field from the rest of the scientific community (Morse, 1999; Morse, Barrett, Mayan, Olson, & Spiers, 2002).

See **Authenticity Criteria, Reliability,** and **Trustworthiness Criteria.**

Variable

A *variable* is an operationalization of a construct.

It may be a 'good' operationalization, in which case the measuring instrument is said to be *valid,* or it may be a 'bad,' or invalid, operationalization. As the name implies, it must be possible to obtain more than one 'score' on that variable; otherwise it would be a constant. Variables that produce a wide spread of scores are especially useful in research, as one of the main objectives is to study how two dimensions 'covary.' If the operationalizations of two constructs do not vary, or vary only slightly, then covariability cannot be properly investigated.

Variables can be classified in several different ways. There are continuous versus discrete variables (a discrete variable that has just two categories is called a dichotomy); 'manifest' versus 'latent' variables (the latter are the constructs themselves); nominal, ordinal, interval, and ratio variables; independent versus dependent variables; antecedent variables, extraneous variables, and mediating variables; and so on. It is the independent versus dependent distinction that is most widely discussed.

Although some authors distinguish between independent and dependent variables only within the context of experimental research, the terms apply equally well to nonexperimental research in which an independent variable is a predictor variable that is supposed to help in explaining the dependent (criterion) variable. However, the independent/dependent distinction breaks down completely in certain studies, for example, factor analytic studies, where all of the variables are on 'equal footing' with one another, that is, none of them is regarded as any sort of cause and none is regarded as any sort of effect.

A common confusion is the labeling of a *category* of a variable as a variable. Stated political preference is a variable; Democrat, Republican, and so on are categories of the variable. Self-reported socioeconomic status is a variable; upper-class, upper-middle class, and so forth are categories of that variable. Statements such as "there is a strong relationship

V

between being a Democrat and being lower-middle class" are methodologically incorrect. Relationships hold between variables, not categories, even though it is the relative frequency of certain combinations of categories that produce those relationships. It is often easier to phrase the research question in terms of relationships between categories than in terms of relationships between variables. For example, "What is the relationship between smoking and lung cancer?" although incorrect, flows more naturally than "What is the relationship between number of cigarettes smoked and amount of lung cancer?"

Example: Although not usually regarded as such, sex is actually a construct. One operationalization of that construct is the self-reporting of one's 'maleness' or 'femaleness.' Because sex is almost always 'measured' this way, the distinction between construct and variable for such dimensions is rarely made, but really should be. Self-report of sex is clearly not the only way to operationalize that construct, and for very young children (especially babies) it is impractical, unreliable, and invalid.

Variance

The *variance* of a set of data for a variable is the mean of the squared deviations (differences) from the mean. It is the square of the standard deviation. Both are measures of dispersion.

See **Standard Deviation.**

Verisimilitude

Verisimilitude is a criterion for judging the quality of a written qualitative research report, in terms of its literary style. A well-written report will "meet literary criteria of coherence, verisimilitude, and interest" through creative, "evocative forms" or *representations that convey plausible 'truths' or realities in ways that make them seem to come alive for the reader (Richardson, 2000, p. 931).

Verstehen

See **Interpretivism.**

Visual Analogue Scale

A *visual analogue scale* is a line that is usually 100 millimeters in length, with descriptive anchors at the ends, and on which additional descriptors are sometimes located. The subject is asked to indicate a point on that line that represents his or her feeling about a particular matter.

Example: In assessing overall attitude toward abortion, a researcher might use a visual analogue scale with the words "It should never be permitted under any circumstance" at one end of the scale and the words

"It should always be permitted under any circumstance" at the other end of the scale. Possible scores for such a scale could range from 0 (for never) to 100 (for always).

Visual analogue scales yield data that can usually be treated as conceptually continuous and therefore amenable for most traditional statistical analyses.

The advantages and disadvantages of visual analogue scales are summarized very nicely by Wewers and Lowe (1990) and by Cline, Herman, Shaw, and Morton (1992).

Elkins, Staniunas, Rajab, Marcus, and Snyder (2004) provide a recent example of the use of a visual analogue scale.

Voice

The concept of *voice* is central to issues of representation in qualitative research reports, that is, (a) the 'voice' used by the researcher and (b) the representation of research participants' 'voices' in these texts. (This also assumes that there are many 'voices' that are part of the sociocultural and personal contexts that are woven into the fabric of researcher interpretations of human experiences.) Lincoln & Guba (2000) illustrate how reporting styles, in terms of 'authorial voice,' may vary across research *paradigms, from the lone 'voice' of the researcher to representational styles featuring the 'mixed voices' of the researcher and research participants. The textual representation of 'mixed voices' is problematic in terms of 'what' and 'whose voices' are heard (or not heard), that is, a matter of 'privileging' certain accounts. Van Maanen's (1988) highly readable and informative text about 'authorial voice' and the rhetorical styles that ethnographers use to present their work helps to sort out different writing strategies that researchers have used to produce valid as well as engaging accounts of their fieldwork.

Intertwined with narrative concerns about how best to 'give voice' to persons are political concerns about who has the authority to do so. Gergen and Gergen (2000) discuss the inclusion of multiple voices within research reports (*multivocality* or *multiple voicing*) as one way to reduce the interpretive "omniscience" of a single authorial voice, but conclude that one of the problems is that the investigator ultimately functions as the "coordinator of the voices" (p. 1028). They offer an ideological view of _polyvocality,_ in the critical mode of post-Marxian and feminist scholarship, as a more effective way to replace the researcher's assumed authority to 'give voice' to participants by equalizing them and thereby establishing a conceptual foundation for new research methodologies that are communally generated. This agenda also serves longstanding concerns about the politics of representation that are common to many researchers who feature the *voices* (actual words and interpreted points

V

189

of view) of research participants who they believe may have been marginalized, excluded, or silenced in current social and political milieus. Feminist researchers, for example, use techniques designed to bring women's 'voices' to the forefront of public arenas where they may have been noticeably absent.

For nursing examples of voicing health concerns, see Haley and Harrigan (2004), Lewis (2004), Semenic, Callister, and Feldman (2004), and Thorne, Con, McGuinness, McPherson, and Harris (2004).

See **Representation.**

V

W

Worldview

Used synonymously with the German *Weltanschauung* ('look onto the world'), in philosophy of science, *worldview* refers to a global pattern of beliefs that, as is true of *paradigms,* constitutes a school of thought and its attendant knowledge claims. Some philosophers (e.g., Feyerabend, Toulmin, Hanson, Kuhn, Foucault) have theorized that the nature and direction of scientific investigation is influenced by the investigator's worldview (Weltanschauung) and is not simply a matter of empirical observation.

The term *worldview* also is used to refer to a particular social or cultural group's outlook on, and beliefs about, its world. These views could include a wide range of generally held notions about the role of the individual in society; how people ought to relate to one another; people's relationship to nature; or the role of kinship, economic, political and religious institutions in the society and in individuals' lives. Some qualitative investigations of an ethnographic, hermeneutic, or historical nature may be particularly interested in examining the worldview of a group of people. However, it is always difficult to know what elements should be incorporated into a description or interpretation of a people's worldview, since individual members of a group will never respond to all the features of the view that is ascribed to them in precisely the same ways.

See **Paradigm.**

W

Z

Zero-Order Correlation Coefficient

A *zero-order correlation coefficient* is a 'Pearson r' that indicates the magnitude and direction of the 'raw' linear relationship between two variables (no 'partialing').

See **Partial Correlation Coefficient** and **Pearson Product-Moment Correlation Coefficient.**

Z

REFERENCES

AbuAlRub, R. F. (2004). Job stress, job performance, and social support among hospital nurses. *Journal of Nursing Scholarship, 36*, 73–78.

Aiken, L. H., Clarke, S. P., Cheung, R. B., Sloane, D. M., & Silber, J. H. (2003). Educational levels of hospital nurses and surgical patient mortality. *JAMA, 290*, 1617–1623.

Allison, P. D. (2001). *Missing data*. Thousand Oaks, CA: Sage.

Altschuld, J. W., & Witkin, B. R. (1999). *From needs assessment to action*. Thousand Oaks, CA: Sage.

American Association for the History of Nursing, Inc. (2001). Position paper. Nursing history in the curriculum: Preparing nurses for the 21st Century. Author. Retrieved March 18, 2005, from http://www.aahn.org/position.html

Anderson, J., Perry, J., Blue, C., Browne, A., Henderson, A., Khan, K. B. et al. (2003). "Rewriting" cultural safety within the postcolonial and postnational feminist project: Toward new epistemologies of healing. *Advances in Nursing Science, 26*(3), 196–214.

Anderson, N. L., Nyamathi, A., McAvoy, J. A., Conde, F., & Casey, C. (2001). Perceptions about risk for HIV/AIDS among adolescents in juvenile detention. *Western Journal of Nursing Research, 23*, 336–359.

Ansari, W. E., Phillips, C. J., & Zwi, A. B. (2004). Public health nurses' perspectives on collaborative partnerships in South Africa. *Public Health Nursing, 21*, 277–286.

Avant, K. C. (2000). The Wilson Method of concept analysis. In B. L. Rodgers & K. A. Knafl (Eds.), *Concept development in nursing: Foundations, techniques, and applications* (pp. 55–76). Philadelphia: W.B. Saunders.

Baggens, C. A. L. (2004). The institution enters the family home: Home visits in Sweden to new parents by the child health care nurse. *Journal of Community Health Nursing, 21*, 15–27.

Bailey, P. H. (2004). The dyspnea-anxiety-dyspnea cycle—COPD patients' stories of breathlessness: "It's scary/When you can't breathe." *Qualitative Health Research, 14*, 760–778.

Barhyte, D., Redman, B. K., & Neill, K. M. (1990). Population or sample: Design decision. *Nursing Research, 39*, 309–310.

Barnum, B. S. (1998). *Nursing theory: Analysis, application, evaluation* (5th ed.). Philadelphia: Lippincott.

Baron, R. M., & Kenny, D. A. (1986). The moderator-mediator variable distinction in social psychological research: Conceptual, strategic, and statistical considerations. *Journal of Personality and Social Psychology, 51*, 1173–1182.

Barthes, R. (1984). *Mythologies*. New York: Hill & Wang.

Barthes, R. (1986). *The rustle of language*. New York: Hill & Wang.

Bashore, L. (2004). Childhood and adolescent cancer survivors' knowledge of their disease and effects of treatment. *Journal of Pediatric Oncology Nursing, 21*, 98–102.

Bates-Jensen, B. M., Cadogan, M., Osterweil, D., Levy-Storms, L., Jorge, J., Al-Samarrai, N., et al. (2003). The minimum data set pressure ulcer indicator: Does it reflect differences in care processes related to pressure ulcer prevention and treatment in nursing homes? *Journal of the American Geriatrics Society, 51*, 1203–1212.

Beck, C. T. (2004). Birth trauma: In the eye of the beholder. *Nursing Research, 5*, 28–35.

References

Beebe, J. (1995). Basic concepts and techniques of rapid appraisal. *Human Organization, 54*(1), 42–51.

Beebe, J. (2001). *Rapid assessment process: An introduction.* Walnut Creek, CA: Alta Mira.

Benner, P. (1983). Uncovering the knowledge embedded in clinical practice. *Image: The Journal of Nursing Scholarship, 19,* 21–34.

Benner, P. (1984). *From novice to expert: Excellence and power in clinical practice.* Menlo Park, CA: Addison-Wesley.

Benner, P. (2000). The roles of embodiment, emotion and lifeworld for rationality and agency in nursing practice. *Nursing Philosophy, 1,* 5–19.

Benner, P., & Tanner, C. (1987). Clinical judgment: How expert nurses use intuition. *American Journal of Nursing, 87,* 23–31.

Benner, P., & Wrubel, J. (1989). *The primacy of caring: Stress and coping in health and illness.* Menlo Park, CA: Addison-Wesley.

Bennett, J. A. (2000). Mediator and moderator variables in nursing research: Conceptual and statistical differences. *Research in Nursing & Health, 23,* 415–420.

Bennett, J. A., Stewart, A. L., Kayser-Jones, J., & Glaser, D. (2002). The mediating effect of pain and fatigue on level of functioning in older adults. *Nursing Research, 51,* 254–265.

Bennett, S. J., Oldridge, N. B., Eckert, G. J., Emblee, J. L., Browning, S., Hou, N., et al. (2003). Comparison of quality of life measures in heart failure. *Nursing Research, 52,* 207–216.

Bent, K. N. (2003). "The people know what they want": An empowerment process of sustainable, ecological community health. *Advances in Nursing Science, 26*(3), 215–226.

Berkhout, A. J. M. B., Boumans, N. P. G., Van Breukelen, G. P. J., Abu-Saad, H. H., & Nijhuis, F. J. N. (2004). Resident-oriented care in nursing homes: Effects on nurses. *Journal of Advanced Nursing, 45,* 621–632.

Bernstein, R. J. (1983). *Beyond objectivism and relativism: Science, hermeneutics, and praxis.* Philadelphia: University of Pennsylvania Press.

Bishop, A. H., & Scudder, J. R. (2003). Gadow's contribution to our philosophical interpretation of nursing. *Nursing Philosophy, 4,* 104–110.

Bliss, D. Z., Fischer, L. R., Savik, K., Avery, M., & Mark, P. (2004). Severity of fecal incontinence in community-living elderly in a health maintenance organization. *Research in Nursing & Health, 27,* 162–173.

Blumer, H. (1969). *Symbolic interaction: Perspective and method.* Englewood Cliffs, NJ: Prentice-Hall.

Börjesson, B., Paperin, C., & Lindell, M. (2004). Maternal support during the first year of infancy. *Journal of Advanced Nursing, 45,* 588–594.

Bowles, C. (1986). Measure of attitude toward menopause using the semantic differential model. *Nursing Research, 35,* 81–85.

Brown, J. K., Porter, L. A., & Knapp, T. R. (1993). The applicability of sequential analysis to nursing research. *Nursing Research, 42,* 280–282.

Browne, A. J. (2000). The potential contributions of critical social theory to nursing science. *Canadian Journal of Nursing Research, 32*(2), 35–55.

Bruce, B. S., Lake, J. P., Eden, V. A., & Denney, J. C. (2004). Children at risk of injury. *Journal of Pediatric Nursing, 19,* 121–127.

Brush, B. L., & Capezuti, E. (2001). Historical analysis of siderail use in American hospitals. *Journal of Nursing Scholarship, 33,* 381–385.

Brush, B. L., Lynaugh, J. E., Boschma, G., Rafferty, A. M., Stuart, M., & Tomes, N. J. (1999). *Nurses of all nations: A history of the International Council of Nurses 1899–1999.* Philadelphia: Lippincott.

Campbell, D. T., & Fiske, D. W. (1959). Convergent and discriminant validation by the multitrait-multimethod matrix. *Psychological Bulletin, 56,* 81–105.

Campbell, D. T., & Stanley, J. C. (1966). *Experimental and quasi-experimental designs for research.* Chicago: Rand McNally.

Canales, M. K., & Geller, B. M. (2004). Moving in between mammography: Screening decisions of American Indian women in Vermont. *Qualitative Health Research, 14,* 836–857.

Cannaerts, N., de Casterlé, M. D., & Grypdonck, M. (2004). Palliative care, care for life: A study of the specificity of residential palliative care. *Qualitative Health Research, 14,* 816–835.

Carlsson, G., Dahlberg, K., Lützen, K., & Nystrom, M. (2004). Violent encounters in psychiatric care: A phenomenological study of embodied caring knowledge. *Issues in Mental Health Nursing, 25,* 191–217.

Caron, C. D., & Bowers, B. J. (2000). Methods and application of dimensional analysis: A contribution to concept and knowledge development in nursing. In B. L. Rodgers & K. A. Knafl (Eds.), *Concept development in nursing: Foundations, techniques, and applications* (2nd ed., pp. 285–319). Philadelphia: W.B. Saunders.

Carper, B. A. (1978). Fundamental patterns of knowing in nursing. *Advances in Nursing Science, 1*(1), 13–23.

Chalmers, K., Gupton, A., Katz, A., Hack, T., Hildes-Ripstein, E., Brown, J., et al. (2004). The description and evaluation of a longitudinal pilot study of a smoking relapse/reduction intervention for perinatal women. *Journal of Advanced Nursing, 45,* 162–171.

Champion, J. D., Shain, R. N., & Piper, J. (2004). Minority adolescent women with sexually transmitted diseases and a history of sexual or physical abuse. *Issues in Mental Health Nursing, 25,* 293–316.

Chang, B. L. (2004). Internet intervention for community elders: Process and feasibility. *Western Journal of Nursing Research, 26,* 461–466.

Charmaz, K. (2000). Grounded theory: Objectivist and constructivist methods. In N. K. Denzin & Y. S. Lincoln (Eds.), *Handbook of qualitative research* (2nd ed., pp. 509–535). Thousand Oaks, CA: Sage.

Chinn, P. L. (1994). Developing a method for aesthetic knowing in nursing. In P. L. Chinn & J. Watson (Eds.), *Art and aesthetics in nursing* (pp. 19–40). New York: National League for Nursing Press.

Chinn, P. L., & Kramer, M. K. (1991/1995). *Theory and nursing: A systematic approach* (3rd & 4th eds.). St. Louis: C.V. Mosby.

Chinn, P. L., & Kramer, M. K. (2004). *Integrated knowledge development in nursing* (6th ed.). St. Louis: C.V. Mosby.

Chinn, P. L., Maeve, M. K., & Bostick, C. (1997). Aesthetic inquiry and the art of nursing. *Scholarly Inquiry for Nursing Practice: An International Journal, 11,* 83–96.

Chiu, L., Emblen, J. D., Hofwegen, L. V., Sawatzky, R., & Meyerhoff, H. (2004). An integrative review of the concept of spirituality in the health sciences. *Western Journal of Nursing Research, 26,* 405–428.

Cho, S-H. (2003). Using multilevel analysis in patient and organizational outcomes research. *Nursing Research, 52,* 61–65.

Cho, S-H., Ketefian, S., Barkauskas, V. H., & Smith, D. G. (2003). The effects of nurse staffing on adverse events, morbidity, mortality, and medical costs. *Nursing Research, 52,* 71–79.

Ciliska, D., DiCenso, A., Melnyk, B. M., & Stetler, C. (2005). Using models and strategies for evidence-based practice. In B. M. Melnyk & E. Fineout-Overholt (Eds.), *Evidence-based practice in nursing and health: A guide to best practice* (pp. 185–219). Philadelphia: Lippincott.

Clark, L., Barton, J. A., & Brown, N. J. (2002). Assessment of community contamination: A critical approach. *Public Health Nursing, 19,* 354–365.

Clarke, S. P. (2004). International collaborations in nursing research: The experience of the International Hospital Outcomes Study. *Applied Nursing Research, 17,* 134–136.

Cline, M., Herman, J., Shaw, E. R., & Morton, R. D. (1992). Standardization of the visual analogue scale. *Nursing Research, 41,* 378–380.

Cody, W. K. (2003). Nursing theory as a guide to practice. *Nursing Science Quarterly, 16,* 225–231.

Cohen, J. (1988). *Statistical power analysis for the behavioral sciences* (2nd ed.). Hillsdale, NJ: Erlbaum.

Cohen, J., Cohen, P., West, S. G., & Aiken, L. S. (2003). *Applied multiple regression/correlation analysis for the behavioral sciences* (3rd ed.). Mahwah, NJ: Erlbaum.

Conn, V. S., & Rantz, M. J. (2003). Research methods: Managing primary study quality in meta-analysis. *Research in Nursing & Health, 26,* 322–333.

Connolly, C. A. (2004). Beyond social history: New approaches to understanding the state of and the state in nursing history. *Nursing History Review, 12,* 5–24.

Cook, T. D., & Campbell, D. T. (1979). *Quasi-experimentation: Design and analysis issues for field settings.* Chicago: Rand McNally.

References

Cotton, A. H. (2003). The discursive field of Web-based health research: Implications for nursing research in cyberspace. *Advances in Nursing Science, 26*(4), 307–319.

Crabtree, S. A. (2003). Asylum blues: Staff attitudes toward psychiatric nursing in Sarawak, East Malaysia. *Journal of Psychiatric and Mental Health Nursing, 10,* 713–721.

Crane, P. B., & McSweeney, J. C. (2004). Informed consent: A process to facilitate older adults' participation in research. *Journal of Gerontological Nursing, 30,* 40–44.

Creedy, D. K., Dennis, C-L., Blyth, R., Moyle, W., Pratt, J., & DeVries, S. M. (2003). Psychometric characteristics of the breastfeeding self-efficacy scale: Data from an Australian sample. *Research in Nursing & Health, 26,* 143–152.

Creswell, J. W. (1998). *Qualitative inquiry and research design: Choosing among five traditions.* Thousand Oaks, CA: Sage.

Creswell, J. W. (2003). *Research design: Qualitative, quantitative, and mixed methods approaches* (2nd ed.). Thousand Oaks, CA: Sage.

Crist, J. D. (2002). Mexican American elders' use of skilled home care nursing services. *Public Health Nursing, 19,* 366–376.

Cronbach, L. J. (1951). Coefficient alpha and the internal structure of tests. *Psychometrika, 16,* 297–334.

Crotty, M. (1998). *The foundations of social research: Meaning and perspective in the research process.* London: Sage.

Dabbs, A. D. V., Hoffman, L. A., Swigart, V., Happ, M. B., Iacono, A. T., & Dauber, J. H. (2004). Using conceptual triangulation to develop an integrated model of the symptom experience of acute rejection after lung transplantation. *Advances in Nursing Science, 27*(2), 138–149.

Darlington, R. B. (1990). *Regression and linear models.* New York: McGraw-Hill.

Daroszewski, E. B. (2004). Commentary by Daroszewski. *Western Journal of Nursing Research, 26,* 170–172.

Davidson, P., Cockburn, J., Daly, J., & Fisher, R. S. (2004). Patient-centered needs assessment: Rationale for a psychometric measure for assessing needs in heart failure. *Journal of Cardiovascular Nursing, 19,* 164–171.

DeKeyser, F. G., & Pugh, L. C. (1990). Assessment of the reliability and validity of biochemical measures. *Nursing Research, 39,* 314–317.

Denzin, N. K. (1989). *Interpretive interactionism.* Newbury Park, CA: Sage.

Denzin, N. K., & Lincoln, Y. S. (2000). Introduction: The discipline and practice of qualitative research. In N. K. Denzin & Y. S. Lincoln (Eds.), *Handbook of qualitative research* (2nd ed., pp. 1–28). Thousand Oaks, CA: Sage.

Devane, D., Begley, C. M., & Clarke, M. (2004). How many do I need? Basic principles of sample size estimation. *Journal of Advanced Nursing, 47,* 297–302.

Dickoff, J., James, P., & Wiedenbach, E. (1968a) Theory in a practice discipline, Part I. *Nursing Research, 17,* 415–435.

Dickoff, J., James, P., & Wiedenbach, E. (1968b). Theory in a practice discipline, Part II. *Nursing Research, 17,* 545–554.

Dickson, G. L. (1990). A feminist poststructuralist analysis of the knowledge of menopause. *Advances in Nursing Science, 12*(3), 15–31.

DiMattio, M. J., & Tulman, L. (2003). A longitudinal study of functional status and correlates following coronary artery bypass graft surgery in women. *Nursing Research, 52,* 98–107.

DiNapoli, P. P. (2003). Guns and dolls: An exploration of violent behavior in girls. *Advances in Nursing Science, 26*(2), 140–148.

Dodgson, J. E., Henly, S. J., Duckett, L., & Tarrant, M. (2003). Theory of planned behavior-based models of breastfeeding duration among Hong Kong mothers. *Nursing Research, 52,* 148–158.

Dombeck, M-T. B. (1996). Chaos and self-organization as a consequence of spiritual disequilibrium. *Clinical Nurse Specialist, 10,* 69–73.

Dombeck, M-T. B. (2003). Work narratives: Gender and race in professional personhood. *Research in Nursing and Health, 26,* 351–365.

Dombeck, M-T. B., Markakis, K., Brachman, L., Dalal, B., & Olsan, T. (2003). Analysis of a biopsychosocial correspondence: Models, mentors, and meanings. In R. M. Frankel, T. E. Quill, & S. H. McDaniel (Eds.), *The biopsychosocial approach: Past, present, future* (pp. 231–251). Rochester, NY: University of Rochester Press.

Dudley, W. N., Benuzillo, J. G., & Carrico, M. S. (2004). SPSS and SAS programming for the testing of mediation models. *Nursing Research, 53,* 59–62.

Dunn, C. M., & Chadwick, G. L. (2002). *Protecting study volunteers in research.* Boston: Thomson Centerwatch.

Dzurec, L. C. (2003). Poststructuralist musings on the mind/body question in health care. *Advances in Nursing Science, 26*(1), 63–76.

Easton, K. L., McComish, J. F., & Greenberg, R. (2000). Avoiding common pitfalls in qualitative data collection and transcription. *Qualitative Health Research, 10,* 703–707.

Edwards, S., & Liaschenko, J. (Eds.). (N.D.) Aims and scope. *Nursing Philosophy.* Retrieved March 18, 2005, from http://www.blackwellpublishing.com/journal.asp?ref=14466-7681&site=1

Eisner, E. (1985). Aesthetic modes of knowing. In E. Eisner (Ed.), *Learning and teaching the ways of knowing: Part II* (pp. 23–36). Chicago: University of Chicago Press.

Elkins, G., Staniunas, R., Rajab, M. H., Marcus, J., & Snyder, T. (2004). Use of a numeric visual analog scale among patients undergoing colorectal surgery. *Clinical Nursing Research, 13,* 237–244.

Elliott, L., Crombie, I. K., Irvine, L., Cantrell, J., & Taylor, J. (2004). The effectiveness of public health nursing: The problems and solutions in carrying out a review of systematic reviews. *Journal of Advanced Nursing, 45,* 117–125.

Endo, E. (2004). Nursing praxis within Margaret Newman's theory of health as expanding consciousness. *Nursing Science Quarterly, 17,* 110–115.

Engstrom, J. L. (1988). Assessment of the reliability of physical measures. *Research in Nursing and Health, 11,* 383–389.

Evidence-Based Medicine Working Group. (1992). Evidence-based medicine: A new approach to teaching the practice of medicine. *JAMA, 268,* 2420–2425.

Eysenck, H. J. (1978). An exercise in mega-silliness. *American Psychologist, 33,* 517.

Fager, J. H., & Melnyk, B. M. (2004). The effectiveness of intervention studies to decrease alcohol use in college undergraduate students: An integrative analysis. *Worldviews on Evidence-Based Nursing, 1,* 102–119.

Fairman, J., & Kagan, S. (1999). Creating critical care: The case of the Hospital of the University of Pennsylvania, 1950–1965. *Advances in Nursing Science, 22*(1), 63–77.

Fairman, J., & Mahon, M. M. (2001). Oral history of Florence Downs: The early years. *Nursing Research, 50,* 322–328.

Fawcett, J. (1984). The metaparadigm of nursing: Present status and future refinements. *Image: Journal of Nursing Scholarship, 16,* 84–87.

Fawcett, J. (2000). *Analysis and evaluation of contemporary nursing knowledge: Nursing models and theories.* Philadelphia: F.A. Davis.

Fawcett, J. (2003a). Theory and practice: A conversation with Marilyn E. Parker. *Nursing Science Quarterly, 16,* 131–136.

Fawcett, J. (2003b). Theory and practice: A discussion with William K. Cody. *Nursing Science Quarterly, 16,* 225–231.

Fawcett, J., Watson, J., Neuman, B., Hinton Walker, P., & Fitzpatrick, J. J. (2001). On nursing theories and evidence. *Journal of Nursing Scholarship, 33,* 115–119.

Fealy, G. M. (2004). 'The good nurse': Visions and values in images of the nurse. *Journal of Advanced Nursing, 46,* 649–656.

Feldman, P. H., & McDonald, M. V. (2004). Conducting translation research in the home care setting: Lessons from a just-in-time reminder study. *Worldviews on Evidence-Based Nursing, 1,* 49–59.

Ferketich, S., & Verran, J. (1986). Exploratory data analysis: Introduction. *Western Journal of Nursing Research, 8,* 464–466.

Field, M. J., Tranquada, R. E., & Feasley, J. C. (Eds.). (1995). *Committee on health services research: Training and work force issues, Institute of Medicine.* Washington, DC: National Academy Press.

Finfgeld, D. L. (2004). Empowerment of individuals with enduring mental health problems: Results from concept analysis and qualitative investigations. *Advances in Nursing Science, 27,* 44–52.

Finney, J. W., Mitchell, R. E., Cronkhite, R. C., & Moos, R. H. (1984). Methodological issues in estimating main and interactive effects: Examples from coping, social support and stress field. *Journal of Health and Social Behavior, 25,* 85–98.

References

Fitzpatrick, J. J., & Whall, A. L. (1996). *Conceptual models of nursing: Analysis and application* (3rd ed.). Norwalk, CT: Appleton & Lange.

Flew, A. (1979). *A dictionary of philosophy.* New York: St. Martin's Press.

Floyd, J. A. (1993). Systematic sampling: Theory and clinical methods. *Nursing Research, 42,* 290–293.

Fontana, J. S. (2004). A methodology for critical science in nursing. *Advances in Nursing Science, 27*(2), 93–101.

Francis, B. (2000). Poststructuralism and nursing: Uncomfortable bedfellows? *Nursing Inquiry, 7,* 20–28.

Frank, A. W. (2004). After methods, the story: From incongruity to truth in qualitative research. *Qualitative Health Research, 14,* 430–440.

Fraser, K. D., & Strang, V. (2004). Decision-making and nurse case management: A philosophical perspective. *Advances in Nursing Science, 27*(1), 32–43.

Gadow, S. (1995a). Clinical epistemology: A dialectic of nursing assessment. *Canadian Journal of Nursing Research, 27,* 25–34.

Gadow, S. (1995b). Narrative and exploration: Toward a poetics of knowledge in nursing. *Nursing Inquiry, 2,* 211–214.

Gadow, S. (1999). Relational narrative: The postmodern turn in nursing ethics. *Scholarly Inquiry in Nursing Practice, 13,* 57–70.

Gadow, S. (2000). Philosophy as falling: Aiming for grace. *Nursing Philosophy, 1,* 89–97.

Gadow, S. (2003). Restorative nursing: Toward a philosophy of postmodern punishment. *Nursing Philosophy, 4,* 161–167.

Geertz, C. (1973). Thick description: Toward an interpretive theory of culture. In C. Geertz, *The interpretation of cultures* (pp. 3–30). New York: Basic Books.

Geertz, C. (1983a). Blurred genres: The refiguration of social thought. In C. Geertz, *Local knowledge: Further essays in interpretive anthropology* (pp. 19–35). New York: Basic Books.

Geertz, C. (1983b). "From the native's point of view": On the nature of anthropological understanding. In C. Geertz, *Local knowledge: Further essays in interpretive anthropology* (pp. 53–70). New York: Basic Books.

Geertz, C. (1983c). Introduction. In C. Geertz, *Local knowledge: Further essays in interpretive anthropology* (pp. 3–16). New York: Basic Books.

Georges, J. M. (2002). Suffering: Toward a contextual praxis. *Advances in Nursing Science, 25*(1), 79–86.

Georges, J. M. (2003). An emerging discourse: Toward epistemic diversity in nursing. *Advances in Nursing Science, 26*(1), 44–52.

Georges, J. M., & McGuire, S. S. (2004). Deconstructing clinical pathways: Mapping the landscape of health care. *Advances in Nursing Science, 27*(1), 2–11.

Gergen, M. M., & Gergen, K. J. (2000). Qualitative inquiry: Tensions and transformations. In N. K. Denzin & Y. S. Lincoln (Eds.), *Handbook of qualitative research* (2nd ed., pp. 1025–1046). Thousand Oaks, CA: Sage.

Gerrish, K., & Griffith, V. (2004). Integration of overseas Registered Nurses: Evaluation of an adaptation programme. *Journal of Advanced Nursing, 45,* 579–587.

Glaser, B. G. (1978). *Theoretical sensitivity.* Mill Valley, CA: Sociology Press.

Glaser, B. G. (1992). *Emergence vs. forcing: Basics of grounded theory analysis.* Mill Valley, CA: Sociology Press.

Glaser, B. G., & Strauss, A. L. (1967). *The discovery of grounded theory: Strategies for qualitative research.* Chicago: Aldine.

Glass, G. V (1976). Primary, secondary, and meta-analysis of research. *Educational Researcher, 5,* 3–8.

Glass, N., & Davis, K. (2004). Reconceptualizing vulnerability: Deconstruction and reconstruction as a postmodern feminist analytical research method. *Advances in Nursing Science, 27*(2), 82–92.

Glazer, S. (2001). Therapeutic touch and postmodernism in nursing. *Nursing Philosophy, 2,* 196–212.

Goffman, E. (1959). *The presentation of self in everyday life.* Garden City, NY: Doubleday Anchor.

Goffman, E. (1967). *Interaction ritual: Essays in face-to-face behavior.* Chicago: Aldine.

Gramling, L. F., & Carr, R. L. (2004). Lifelines: A life history methodology. *Nursing Research, 53,* 207–210.

Green, S., Benedetti, J., & Crowley, J. (2002). *Clinical trials in oncology* (2nd ed.). New York: Chapman & Hall.

Greenwood, D. J., & Levin, M. (2000) Reconstructing the relationships between universities and society through action research. In N. K. Denzin & Y. S. Lincoln (Eds.), *Handbook of qualitative research* (2nd ed., pp. 85–106). Thousand Oaks, CA: Sage.

Guba, E. G., & Lincoln, Y. S. (1989). *Fourth generation evaluation*. Newbury Park, CA: Sage.

Guba, E. G., & Lincoln, Y. S. (1994). Competing paradigms in qualitative research. In N. K. Denzin & Y. S. Lincoln (Eds.), *Handbook of qualitative research* (pp. 105–117). Thousand Oaks, CA: Sage.

Gubrium, J. F., & Holstein, J. A. (2000). Analyzing interpretive practice. In N. K. Denzin & Y. S. Lincoln (Eds.), *Handbook of qualitative research* (2nd ed., pp. 487–508). Thousand Oaks, CA: Sage.

Guttman, L. (1941). The quantification of a class of attributes: A theory and method for scale construction. In P. Horst (Ed.), *The prediction of personal adjustment* (pp. 251–364). New York: Social Science Research Council.

Guyatt, G., & Rennie, D. (2002). *Users' guides to the medical literature: Essentials of evidence-based clinical practice*. Chicago, IL: AMA Press

Haase, J. E., Leidy, N. K., Coward, D. D., Britt, T., & Penn, P. E. (2000). Simultaneous Concept Analysis: A strategy for developing multiple interrelated concepts. In B. L. Rodgers & K. A. Knafl (Eds.), *Concept development in nursing: Foundations, techniques, and applications* (pp. 209–229). Philadelphia: W.B. Saunders.

Haley, J., & Harrigan, R. C. (2004). Voicing the strengths of Pacific Island parent caregivers of children who are medically fragile. *Journal of Transcultural Nursing, 15,* 184–194.

Hall, J. E. (2004). Pluralistic evaluation: A situational approach to service evaluation. *Journal of Nursing Management, 12,* 22–27.

Halpern, E. S. (1983). *Auditing naturalistic inquiries: The development and application of a model*. Unpublished doctoral dissertation, Indiana University.

Hamilton, D. B. (1993). The idea of history and the history of ideas. *Image, 18,* 53–57.

Hanley, J. A., Negassa, A., Edwardes, M. D. deB., & Forrester, J. E. (2003). Statistical analysis of correlated data using generalized estimating equations: An orientation. *American Journal of Epidemiology, 157,* 364–375. [See also the letters regarding this article by Godbold and by Zou, and Hanley's reply (*American Journal of Epidemiology, 158,* 289–290).]

Hardin, J. W., & Hilbe, J. M. (2003). *Generalized estimating equations*. Boca Raton, FL: Chapman & Hall/CRC.

Hardin, P. K. (2003). Social and cultural considerations in recovery from anorexia nervosa. *Advances in Nursing Science, 26*(1), 5–16.

Hardy, D. J., O'Brien, A. P., Gaskin, C. J., O'Brien, A. J., Morrison-Ngatai, E., Skews, G., et al. (2004). Practical application of the Delphi technique in a bicultural mental health nursing study in New Zealand. *Journal of Advanced Nursing, 46,* 95–109.

Harrington, C., Woolhandler, S., Mullan, J., Carrillo, H., & Himmelstein, D. U. (2001). Does investor ownership of nursing homes compromise the quality of care? *American Journal of Public Health, 91,* 1452–1455.

Hawkes, T. (1977). *Structuralism and semiotics*. Berkeley: University of California Press.

Hebdige, D. (1979). *Subculture: The meaning of style*. London: Methuen.

Hendel, T., Fradkin, M., & Kidron, D. (2004). Physical restraint use in health care settings: Public attitudes in Israel. *Journal of Gerontological Nursing, 30*(2), 12–19.

Herrington, C. J., Olomu, I. N., & Geller, S. M. (2004). Salivary cortisol as indicators of pain in preterm infants. *Clinical Nursing Research, 13,* 53–68.

Higgins, P. A., & Moore, S. M. (2000). Levels of theoretical thinking in nursing. *Nursing Outlook, 48,* 179–183.

Hildebrand, D. L. (2002). *Beyond realism and anti-realism: John Dewey and the neopragmatists*. Nashville, TN: Vanderbilt University Press.

Hinton Walker, P., & Neuman, B. (Eds.). (1996). *Blueprint for use of nursing models: Education, research, practice & administration*. New York: National League for Nursing Press.

Hitchcock, J. M., & Wilson, H. S. (1992). Personal risking: Lesbian self-disclosure of sexual orientation to professional health care providers. *Nursing Research, 41,* 178–183.

Holmes, C. A., & Warelow, P. J. (2000). Some implications of postmodernism for nursing theory, research, and practice. *Canadian Journal of Nursing Research, 32*(2), 89–101.

References

Holsti, O. R. (1969). *Content analysis for the social sciences and humanities.* Reading, MA: Addison-Wesley.

Houweling, L. (2004). Image, function, and style: A history of the nursing uniform. *American Journal of Nursing, 104*(4), 40–48.

Hudson, A., Kirksey, K., & Holzemer, W. (2004). The influence of symptoms on quality of life among HIV-infected women. *Western Journal of Nursing Research, 26,* 9–23.

Hupcey, J. E., & Penrod, J. (2003). Concept advancement: Enhancing inductive validity. *Research and Theory for Nursing Practice: An International Journal, 17,* 19–30.

Hurst, I. (2004). Imposed burdens: A Mexican American mother's experience of family resources in a newborn intensive-care unit. *JOGNN, 33,* 156–163.

Ingersoll, G. L. (1998). Administrative issues in the measurement and management of outcomes. *Applied Nursing Research, 11,* 93–97.

Ingersoll, G. L. (2005). Generating evidence through outcomes management. In B. M. Melnyk & E. Fineout-Overholt (Eds.), *Evidence-based practice in nursing & healthcare* (pp. 299–332). Philadelphia: Lippincott.

Janesick, V. J. (2000). The choreography of qualitative research design: Minuets, improvisations, and crystallization. In N. K. Denzin & Y. S. Lincoln (Eds.), *Handbook of qualitative research* (2nd ed., pp. 379–399). Thousand Oaks, CA: Sage.

Janke, J. (1994). Development of the breast-feeding attrition prediction tool. *Nursing Research, 43,* 100–104.

Jansen, D. A., & von Sadovszky, V. (2004). Restorative activities of community-dwelling elders. *Western Journal of Nursing Research, 26,* 381–399.

Jennings, B. M. (2004). The intersection of nursing administration research and health services research. *JONA: The Journal of Nursing Administration, 34,* 213–215.

Johnston, L. (2005). Critically appraising quantitative evidence. In B. M. Melnyk & E. Fineout-Overholt (Eds.), *Evidence-based practice in nursing & healthcare: A guide to best practice* (pp. 79–125). Philadelphia: Lippincott.

Kaasalainen, S., & Crook, J. (2004). An exploration of seniors' ability to report pain. *Clinical Nursing Research, 13,* 199–215.

Kaplan, A. (1964). *The conduct of inquiry.* New York: Thomas Y. Crowell.

Kayser-Jones, J. (2002). The experience of dying: An ethnographic nursing home study. *The Gerontologist, 42 Spec. No.3,* 11–19.

Kearney, M. H. (1998). Ready-to-wear: Discovering grounded formal theory. *Research in Nursing & Health, 21,* 179–186.

Kearney, M. H. (2001a). Enduring love: A grounded formal theory of women's experience of domestic violence. *Research in Nursing & Health, 24,* 270–282.

Kearney, M. H. (2001b). Levels and applications of qualitative research evidence. *Research in Nursing & Health, 24,* 145–153.

Kearney, M. H., Munro, B. H., Kelly, U., & Hawkins, J. W. (2004). Health behaviors as mediators for the effect of partner abuse on infant birth weight. *Nursing Research, 53,* 36–45.

Keeling, A. W., & Ramos, M. C. (1995). The role of nursing history in preparing nurses for the future. *Nursing & Health Care, 16*(1), 30–34.

Kemmis, S., & McTaggart, R. (2000). Participatory action research. In N. K. Denzin & Y. S. Lincoln (Eds.), *Handbook of qualitative research* (2nd ed., pp. 567–605). Thousand Oaks, CA: Sage.

Kendall, J., Hatton, D., Beckett, A., & Leo, M. (2003). Children's accounts of attention-deficit/hyperactivity disorder. *Advances in Nursing Science, 26*(2), 114–130.

Kidd, L. I., & Tusaie, K. R. (2004). Disconfirming beliefs: The use of poetry to know the lived experience of student nurses in mental health clinicals. *Issues in Mental Health Nursing, 25,* 403–414.

Kiecolt, K. J., & Nathan, L. E. (1985). *Secondary analysis of survey data.* Newbury Park, CA: Sage.

Kikuchi, J. F. (2003). Nursing knowledge and the problem of worldviews. *Research and Theory for Nursing: An International Journal, 17,* 7–17.

Kikuchi, J. F. (2004). Towards a philosophic theory of nursing. *Nursing Philosophy, 5,* 79–83.

Kim, H. S. (2000). *The nature of theoretical thinking in nursing* (2nd ed.). New York: Springer.

Kim, K. H., Sobal, J., & Wethington, E. (2003). Religion and body weight. *International Journal of Obesity, 27,* 469–477.

Kim, S. S. (2004). The experiences of young Korean immigrants: A grounded theory of negotiating social, cultural, and generational boundaries. *Issues in Mental Health Nursing, 25,* 517–537.

Kincheloe, J. L., & McLaren, P. (2000). Rethinking critical theory and qualitative research. In N. K. Denzin & Y. S. Lincoln (Eds.), *Handbook of qualitative research* (2nd ed., pp. 279–313). Thousand Oaks, CA: Sage.

King, K. B., Quinn, J. R., Delehanty, J. M., Rizzo, S., Eldredge, D. H., Caulfield, L., et al. (2002). Perception of risk for coronary heart disease in women undergoing coronary angiography. *Heart & Lung, 31,* 246–252.

Kirkham, S. R., & Anderson, J. M. (2002). Postcolonial nursing scholarship: From epistemology to method. *Advances in Nursing Science, 25*(1), 1–17.

Knafl, K. A., & Deatrick, J. A. (2000). Knowledge synthesis and concept development in nursing. In B. L. Rodgers & K. A., Knafl (Eds.), *Concept development in nursing: Foundations, techniques, and applications* (2nd ed., pp. 39–54). Philadelphia: W.B. Saunders.

Knapp, T. R. (1978). Canonical correlation analysis: A general parametric significance testing system. *Psychological Bulletin, 85,* 410–416.

Knapp, T. R. (1985). Validity, reliability, and neither. *Nursing Research, 34,* 189–192.

Knapp, T. R. (1991). Coefficient alpha: Conceptualizations and anomalies. *Research in Nursing & Health, 14,* 457–460.

Knapp, T. R. (1992). The dilemma of -ic versus -ical. *Nursing Research, 41,* 319.

Knapp, T. R. (1994). Regression analyses: What to report. *Nursing Research, 43,* 187–189.

Knapp, T. R. (1998). *Quantitative nursing research.* Thousand Oaks, CA: Sage.

Knapp, T. R. (2005). *The reliability of measuring instruments* (3rd ed.). Vancouver, BC, Canada: Edgeworth Laboratory for Quantitative Educational and Behavioral Science Series. http://www.educ.ubc.ca/faculty/zumbo/series/knapp/index.htm

Koch, T. (1994). Establishing rigour in qualitative research: The decision trail. *Journal of Advanced Nursing, 19,* 976–986.

Koniak-Griffin, D., Lesser, J., Uman, G., & Nyamathi, A. (2003). Teen pregnancy, motherhood, and unprotected sexual activity. *Research in Nursing & Health, 26,* 4–19.

Koniak-Griffin, D., Verzemnieks, I. L., Anderson, N. L. R., Brecht, M-L., Lesser, J., Kim, S., et al. (2003). Nurse visitation for adolescent mothers. *Nursing Research, 52,* 127–136.

Kools, S., McCarthy, M., Durham, R., & Robrecht, L. (1996). Dimensional analysis: Broadening the conception of grounded theory. *Qualitative Health Research, 6,* 312–330.

Kozuki, Y., & Kennedy, M. G. (2004). Cultural incommensurability in psychodynamic psychotherapy in Western and Japanese traditions. *Journal of Nursing Scholarship, 36,* 30–38.

Kramer, M. K. (2002). Academic talk about dementia caregiving: A critical comment on language. *Research and Theory for Nursing Practice: An International Journal, 16,* 263–280.

Krippendorff, K. (1980). *Content analysis.* Beverly Hills, CA: Sage.

Krueger, R., & Casey, M. A. (2000). *Focus groups: A practical guide for applied research* (3rd ed.). Thousand Oaks, CA: Sage.

Kushner, K. E., & Morrow, R. (2003). Grounded theory, feminist theory, critical theory: Toward theoretical triangulation. *Advances in Nursing Science, 26*(1), 30–43.

Kwak, C., & Clayton-Matthews, A. (2002). Multinomial logistic regression. *Nursing Research, 51,* 404–410.

Lachin, J. M. (1981). Introduction to sample size determination and power analysis for clinical trials. *Controlled Clinical Trials, 2,* 93–113.

LaCoursiere, S. (2003). Research methodology for the internet: External validity (generalizability). *Advances in Nursing Science, 26*(4), 257–273.

Ladson-Billings, G. (2000). Racialized discourses and ethnic epistemologies. In N. K. Denzin & Y. S. Lincoln (Eds.), *Handbook of qualitative research* (2nd ed., pp. 257–277). Thousand Oaks, CA: Sage.

Landis, C. A., Frey, C. A., Lentz, M. J., Rothermel, J., Buchwald, D., & Shaver, J. L. F. (2003). Self-reported sleep quality and fatigue correlates with actigraphy in midlife women with fibromyalgia. *Nursing Research, 52,* 140–147.

Last, J. M. (Ed.). (1995). *A dictionary of epidemiology* (3rd ed.). New York: Oxford University Press.

Leidy, N. K., & Weissfield, L. A. (1991). Sample sizes and power computation for clinical intervention trials. *Western Journal of Nursing Research, 13,* 138–144.

References

Leight, S. B. (2002). Starry night: Using story to inform aesthetic knowing in women's health nursing. *Journal of Advanced Nursing, 37,* 108–114.

Levy, P. S., & Lemeshow, S. (1999). *Sampling of populations: Methods and applications.* New York: Wiley.

Lewis, L. M. (2004). Culturally appropriate substance abuse treatment for parenting African American women. *Issues in Mental Health Nursing, 25,* 451–472.

Li, H. C. W., & Lopez, V. (2004). Psychometric evaluation of the Chinese version of the State Anxiety Scale for children. *Research in Nursing & Health, 27,* 198–207.

Li, H., Melnyk, B. M., McCann, R., Chatcheydang, J., Koulouglioti, C., Nichols, L. W., et al. (2003). Creating avenues for relative empowerment (CARE): A pilot test of an intervention to improve outcomes of hospitalized elders and family caregivers. *Research in Nursing & Health, 26,* 284–299.

Liehr, P., & Smith, M. J. (1999). Middle range theory: Spinning research and practice to create knowledge for the new millennium. *Advances in Nursing Science, 21*(4), 81–91.

Likert, R. (1932). A technique for the measurement of attitudes. *Archives of Psychology, 22,* 5–55.

Lincoln, Y. S., & Denzin, N. K. (2000). The seventh moment: Out of the past. In Y. S. Lincoln & N. K. Denzin (Eds.), *Handbook of qualitative research* (2nd ed., pp. 1047–1065). Thousand Oaks, CA: Sage.

Lincoln, Y. S., & Guba, E. G. (1985). *Naturalistic inquiry.* Beverly Hills, CA: Sage.

Lincoln, Y. S., & Guba, E. G. (2000). Paradigmatic controversies, contradictions, and emerging confluences. In N. K. Denzin & Y. S. Lincoln (Eds.), *Handbook of qualitative research* (2nd ed., pp. 163–188). Thousand Oaks, CA: Sage.

Lindley, P., & Walker, S. N. (1993). Theoretical and methodological differentiation of moderation and mediation. *Nursing Research, 42,* 276–279.

Little, R. J. A., & Rubin, D. B. (2002). *Statistical analysis with missing data* (2nd ed.). New York: Wiley.

Long, K. R., Ritter, P. L., & Gonzalez, V. M. (2003). Hispanic chronic disease self-management. *Nursing Research, 52,* 361–369.

Lorber, J. (2001). *Gender inequality: Feminist theories and politics* (2nd ed.). Los Angeles, CA: Roxbury.

Lucas, M. D., Atwood, J. R., & Hagaman, R. (1993). Replication and validation of Anticipated Turnover Model for urban registered nurses. *Nursing Research, 42,* 184–186.

MacLean, L. M., Meyer, M., & Estable, A. (2004). Improving accuracy of transcripts in qualitative research. *Qualitative Health Research, 14,* 113–123.

Madigan, E. A., Tullai-McGuinness, S., & Fortinsky, R. H. (2003). Accuracy in the outcomes and assessment information set (OASIS): Results of a video simulation. *Research in Nursing & Health, 26,* 273–283.

Madsen, W. (2003). Working for herself: Case study of a private duty nurse. *International History of Nursing Journal, 7*(3), 23–31.

Mahon, N. E., Yarcheski, A., & Yarcheski, T. J. (2004). Social support and positive health practices in early adolescents: A test of mediating variables. *Clinical Nursing Research, 13,* 216–236.

Maxton, F. J. C., Justin, L., & Gillies, D. (2004). Estimating core temperature in infants and children after cardiac surgery: A comparison of six methods. *Journal of Advanced Nursing, 45,* 214–222.

Maxwell, J. A. (1992). Understanding and validity in qualitative research. *Harvard Educational Review, 62,* 279–299.

Maxwell, J. A. (2004). Causal explanation, qualitative research, and scientific inquiry. *Educational Researcher, 33*(2), 3–11.

McCall, W. A. (1939). *Measurement.* New York: MacMillan.

McCarthy, M. C. (2003a). Detecting acute confusion in older adults: Comparing clinical reasoning of nurses working in acute, long-term, and community health care environments. *Research in Nursing & Health, 26,* 203–212.

McCarthy, M. C. (2003b). Situated clinical reasoning: Distinguishing acute confusion from dementia in hospitalized older adults. *Research in Nursing & Health, 26,* 90–101.

McCarthy, P., Chammas, G., Wilimas, J., Alaoui, F. M., & Harif, M. (2004). Managing children's cancer pain in Morocco. *Journal of Nursing Scholarship, 36,* 11–15.

McDonald, D. D., Frakes, M., Apostolidis, B., Armstrong, B., Goldblatt, S., & Bernardo, D. (2003). Effect of a psychiatric diagnosis on nursing care for nonpsychiatric problems. *Research in Nursing & Health, 26,* 225–232.

McErlean, J. (2000). *Philosophies of science: From foundations to contemporary issues.* Belmont, CA: Wadsworth.

McEwen, M., & Wills, E. M. (2002). *Theoretical basis for nursing.* Philadelphia: Lippincott.

McFarlane, J., Malecha, A., Gist, J., Watson, K., Batten, E., Hall, I., et al. (2002). An intervention to increase safety behaviors of abused women. *Nursing Research, 51,* 347–354.

McFarlane, J., Malecha, A., Gist, J., Watson, K., Batten, E., Hall, I., et al. (2004). Increasing the safety-promoting behaviors of abused women. *American Journal of Nursing, 104*(3), 40–50.

McInnes, E., & Askie, L. (2004). Evidence review on older people's views and experiences of falls prevention strategies. *Worldviews on Evidence-Based Nursing, 1,* 20–37.

McIntyre, M. (2003). Cultivating a worldly response: The contribution of Sally Gadow's work to interpretive inquiry. *Nursing Philosophy, 4,* 111–120.

McLaughlin, F. E., & Marascuilo, L. A. (1990). *Advanced nursing and health care research: Quantification approaches.* Philadelphia: W.B. Saunders.

Mead, G. H. (1934). *Mind, self, and society.* Chicago: University of Chicago Press.

Mead, G. H. (1938). *The philosophy of the act.* Chicago: University of Chicago Press.

Mead, G. H. (1959). *The philosophy of the present.* Seattle, WA: Open Court.

Meehan, T. C. (2003). Careful nursing: A model for contemporary nursing practice. *Journal of Advanced Nursing, 44,* 99–107.

Melchior, F. (2004). Feminist approaches to nursing history. *Western Journal of Nursing Research, 26,* 340–355.

Meleis, A. (1997). *Theoretical nursing: Development and progress* (3rd ed.). Philadelphia: J. B. Lippincott.

Melnyk, B. M. (2003). Critical appraisal of systematic reviews: A key strategy for evidence-based practice. *Pediatric Nursing, 29,* 125, 147–149.

Melnyk, B. M., & Fineout-Overholt, E. (Eds.). (2005). *Evidence-based practice in nursing & healthcare: A guide to best practice.* Philadelphia: Lippincott.

Menard, S. (1995). *Applied logistic regression analysis.* Thousand Oaks, CA: Sage.

Meretoja, R., Isoaho, H., & Leino-Kilpi, H. (2004). Nurse competence scale: Development and psychometric testing. *Journal of Advanced Nursing, 47,* 124–133.

Merritt-Gray, M., & Wuest, J. (1995). Counteracting abuse and breaking free: The process of leaving revealed through women's voices. *Health Care for Women International, 16,* 399–412.

Minardi, H. A., & Blanchard, M. (2004). Older people with depression: A pilot study. *Journal of Advanced Nursing, 46,* 23–32.

Minicucci, D. S., Schmitt, M. H., Dombeck, M. T., & Williams, G. C. (2003). Actualizing Gadow's moral framework for nursing through research. *Nursing Philosophy, 4,* 92–103.

Mishel, M. H. (1990). Reconceptualization of the uncertainty in illness theory. *Image: Journal of Nursing Scholarship, 22,* 256–262.

Mitchell, G. J., & Cody, W. K. (1992). Nursing knowledge and human science: Ontological and epistemological considerations. *Nursing Science Quarterly, 5,* 54–61.

Mohr, W. K. (2004). Surfacing the life phases of a mental health support group. *Qualitative Health Research, 14,* 61–77.

Montbriand, M. J. (2004a). Seniors' life histories and perceptions of illness. *Western Journal of Nursing Research, 26,* 242–260.

Montbriand, M. J. (2004b). Seniors' survival trajectories and the illness connection. *Qualitative Health Research, 14,* 449–461.

Morse, J. M. (1998a). Validity by committee. *Qualitative Health Research, 8,* 443–445.

Morse, J. M. (1998b). What's wrong with random selection? *Qualitative Health Research, 8,* 733–735.

Morse, J. M. (1999). Myth #93: Reliability and validity are not relevant to qualitative inquiry. *Qualitative Health Research, 9,* 717.

Morse, J. M. (2000). Determining sample size. *Qualitative Health Research, 10,* 3–5.

Morse, J. M., Barrett, M., Mayan, M., Olson, K., & Spiers, J. (2002). Verification strategies for establishing reliability and validity in qualitative research. *International Journal of Qualitative Methods, 1*(2), pp. 1–10. Retrieved March 15, 2005, from http://www.ualberta.ca/~ijqm.

References

Mueller, M-R. (2004). Clinical, technical, and social contingencies and the decisions of adults with HIV/AIDS to enroll in clinical trials. *Qualitative Health Research, 14,* 704–713.

Munhall, P. L. (1994). *Revisioning phenomenology: Nursing and health science research.* New York: National League for Nursing Press.

Munro, B. H. (2001). *Statistical methods for health care research* (4th ed.). Philadelphia: Lippincott, Williams, & Wilkins.

Murphy, S. A., Chung, I-J., & Johnson, L. C. (2002). Patterns of mental distress following the violent death of a child and predictors of change over time. *Research in Nursing & Health, 25,* 425–437.

Norbeck, J. S. (1981). Social support: A model for clinical research and application. *Advances in Nursing Science, 3*(4), 43–59.

Norris, A. E., & Aroian, K. J. (2004). To transform or not transform skewed data for psychometric analysis—That is the question! *Nursing Research, 53,* 67–71.

Norton, S. A., & Bowers, B. J. (2001). Working toward consensus: Providers' strategies to shift patients from curative to palliative treatment choices. *Research in Nursing and Health, 24,* 258–269.

Okasha, S. (2002). *Philosophy of science: A very short introduction.* Oxford, England: Oxford University Press.

Olade, R. A. (2004). Strategic collaborative model for evidence-based nursing practice. *Worldviews on Evidence-Based Practice, 1,* 60–68.

Olesen, V. L. (2000). Feminisms and qualitative research at and into the millennium. In N. K. Denzin & Y. S. Lincoln (Eds.), *Handbook of qualitative research* (2nd ed., pp. 215–255). Thousand Oaks, CA: Sage.

Olshansky, E. F. (1996). Theoretical issues in building a grounded theory: Application of an example of a program of research on infertility. *Qualitative Health Research, 6,* 394–405.

Olshansky, E. (2003). A theoretical explanation for previously infertile mothers' vulnerability to depression. *Journal of Nursing Scholarship, 35,* 263–268.

Osgood, C. E., Suci, G. H., & Tannenbaum, P. H. (1957). *The measurement of meaning.* Urbana: University of Illinois Press.

Paley, J. (2002). Virtues of autonomy: The Kantian ethics of care. *Nursing Philosophy, 3,* 133–143.

Paley, J. (2004). Gadow's romanticism: Science, poetry, and embodiment in postmodern nursing. *Nursing Philosophy, 5,* 112–126.

Parker, B., Steeves, R., Anderson, S., & Moran, B. (2004). Uxoricide: A phenomenological study of adult survivors. *Issues in Mental Health Nursing, 25,* 133–145.

Parker, M. (2001). *Nursing theories and nursing practice.* Philadelphia: F.A. Davis.

Pedhazur, E. J. (1997). *Multiple regression in behavioral research* (3rd ed.). New York: Holt, Rinehart, & Winston.

Perry, J. (2002). Wives giving care to husbands with Alzheimer's disease: A process of interpretive caring. *Research in Nursing & Health, 25,* 307–316.

Pfeil, M. (2003). The skills-teaching myth in nurse education: From Florence Nightingale to Project 2000. *International History of Nursing Journal, 7*(3), 32–40.

Phillips, D. A., & Drevdahl, D. J. (2003). "Race" and the difficulties of language. *Advances in Nursing Science, 26*(1), 17–29.

Plach, S. K., Stevens, P. E., & Moss, V. A. (2004). Corporeality: Women's experiences of a body with rheumatoid arthritis. *Clinical Nursing Research, 13,* 137–155.

Polit, D. F., & Beck, C. T. (2004). *Nursing research: Principles and methods* (7th ed.). Philadelphia: Lippincott, Williams, & Wilkins.

Polivka, B. J., & Nickel, J. T. (1992). Case-control design: An appropriate strategy for nursing research. *Nursing Research, 41,* 250–253.

Porter, M. L., & Bean, J. P. (2004). Organizational lifecycle in a school of nursing. *Western Journal of Nursing Research, 26,* 444–460.

Powers, B. A. (2001). Ethnographic analysis of everyday ethics in the care of nursing home residents with dementia. *Nursing Research, 50,* 332–339.

Powers, B. A. (2003a). *Nursing home ethics: Everyday issues affecting residents with dementia.* New York: Springer.

Powers, B. A. (2003b). The significance of losing things for nursing home residents with dementia and their families. *Journal of Gerontological Nursing, 29*(11), 43–52.

Powers, B. A. (2005a). Critically appraising qualitative evidence. In B. M. Melnyk & E. Fineout-Overholt (Eds.), *Evidence-based practice in nursing and healthcare: A guide to best practice* (pp. 127–162). Philadelphia: Lippincott.

Powers, B. A. (2005b). Looking for best evidence: "A rose by any other name . . ." In B. M. Melnyk & E. Fineout-Overholt (Eds.), *Evidence-based practice in nursing and healthcare: A guide to best practice* (pp. 547–555). Philadelphia: Lippincott.

Powers, P. (2003). Empowerment as treatment and the role of health professionals. *Advances in Nursing Science, 26*(3), 227–237.

Prescott, P. A., & Soeken, K. L. (1989). The potential uses of pilot work. *Nursing Research, 38,* 60–62.

Prigogine, L., & Stengers, L. (1984). *Order out of chaos: Man's new dialogue with nature.* New York: Bantam Books.

Procter, S., Wilcockson, J., Pearson, P., & Allgar, V. (2001). Going home from hospital: The carer/patient dyad. *Journal of Advanced Nursing, 35,* 206–217.

Puntillo, K., & Weiss, S. J. (1994). Pain: Its mediators and associated morbidity in critically ill cardiovascular surgical patients. *Nursing Research, 43,* 31–36.

Rabinow, P., & Sullivan, W. M. (1979). The interpretive turn: A second look. In P. Rabinow & W. M. Sullivan (Eds.), *Interpretive social science: A second look* (pp. 1–30). Berkeley: University of California Press.

Raudenbush, S. W., & Bryk, A. S. (2002). *Hierarchical linear models* (2nd ed.). Thousand Oaks, CA: Sage.

Reed, P. G. (1995). A treatise on nursing knowledge development for the 21st century: Beyond postmodernism. *Advances in Nursing Science, 17*(3), 70–84.

Reinhardt, A. C. (2004). Discourse on the transformational leader metanarrative or finding the right person for the job. *Advances in Nursing Science, 27*(1), 21–31.

Reynolds, N. R., Timmerman, G., Anderson, J., & Stevenson, J. S. (1992). Meta-analysis for descriptive research. *Research in Nursing & Health, 15,* 467–475.

Richards, L. (1998). Closeness to data: The changing goals of qualitative data handling. *Qualitative Health Research, 8,* 319–328.

Richardson, L. (1994). Writing: A method of inquiry. In N. K. Denzin & Y. S. Lincoln (Eds.), *Handbook of qualitative research* (pp. 516–529). Thousand Oaks, CA: Sage.

Richardson, L. (2000). Writing: A method of inquiry. In N. K. Denzin & Y. S. Lincoln (Eds.), *Handbook of qualitative research* (2nd ed., pp. 923–948). Thousand Oaks, CA: Sage.

Ridner, S. (2004). Psychological distress: Concept analysis. *Journal of Advanced Nursing, 45,* 536–545.

Rizzuto, C., Bostrom, J., Suter, W. N., & Chenitz, W. C. (1994). Predictors of nurses' involvement in research activities. *Western Journal of Nursing Research, 16,* 219–226.

Roberts, S., & Neuringer, A. (1998). Self-experimentation. In K. A. Lattal & M. Perrone (Eds.), *Handbook of research methods in human operant behavior* (pp. 619–655). New York: Plenum.

Robinson, A., & Street, A. (2004). Improving networks between acute care nurses and an aged care assessment team. *Journal of Clinical Nursing, 13,* 486–496.

Rodgers, B. L. (1989). Concept analysis and the development of nursing knowledge: The evolutionary cycle. *Journal of Advanced Nursing, 14,* 330–335.

Rodgers, B. L. (2000). Concept analysis: An evolutionary view. In B. L. Rodgers & K. A. Knafl (Eds.), *Concept development in nursing: Foundations, techniques, and applications* (2nd ed., pp. 77–102). Philadelphia: W.B. Saunders.

Rodgers, B. L., & Cowles, K. V. (1993). The qualitative research audit trail: A complex collection of documentation. *Research in Nursing & Health, 16,* 219–226.

Rodgers, B. L., & Knafl, K. A. (Eds.). (2000). *Concept development in nursing: Foundations, techniques, and applications* (2nd ed.). Philadelphia: W.B. Saunders.

Romyn, D. M. (2000). Emancipatory pedagogy in nursing education: A dialectical analysis. *Canadian Journal of Nursing Research, 32*(2), 119–138.

Rosengren, K. E. (1981). *Advances in content analysis.* Beverly Hills, CA: Sage.

Roth, P. A. (2000). How narratives explain. In J. McErlean (Ed.), *Philosophies of science: From foundations to contemporary issues* (pp. 359–368). Belmont, CA: Wadsworth.

Rowe, M. A., & Fehrenbach, N. (2004). Injuries sustained by community-dwelling individuals with dementia. *Clinical Nursing Research, 13,* 98–110.

References

Rycroft-Malone, J., & Stetler, C. B. (2004). Commentary on evidence, research, knowledge: A call for conceptual clarity: Shannon Scott-Findlay & Carolee Pollock. *Worldviews on Evidence-Based Nursing, 1,* 98–101.

Sackett, D. L., Straus, S. E., Richardson, W. S., Rosenberg, W., & Haynes, R. B. (2000). *Evidence-based medicine* (2nd ed.). Edinburgh, Scotland: Churchill Livingstone.

Sahai, H., & Khurshid, A. (1996). *Statistics in epidemiology: Methods, techniques, and applications.* Boca Raton, FL: CRC Press.

Salazar, M. K., Napolitano, M., Schere, J. A., & McCauley, L. A. (2004). Hispanic adolescent farmworkers' perceptions associated with pesticide exposure and Response [to commentaries]. *Western Journal of Nursing Research, 26,* 146–166, 173–175.

Sandelowski, M. (1993). Rigor or rigor mortis: The problem of rigor in qualitative research revisited. *Research in Nursing & Health, 16,* 1–8.

Sandelowski, M. (1995). Sample size in qualitative research. *Research in Nursing & Health, 18,* 179–183.

Sandelowski, M. (1998). The call to experts in qualitative research. *Research in Nursing & Health, 21,* 467–471.

Sandelowski, M. (1999). Troubling distinctions: A semiotics of the nursing/technology relationship. *Nursing Inquiry, 6,* 198–207.

Sandelowski, M. (2000). Whatever happened to qualitative description? *Research in Nursing & Health, 23,* 334–340.

Sandelowski, M. (2002). Keynote address: Second Annual Advances in Qualitative Methods Conference. Reembodying qualitative inquiry. *Qualitative Health Research, 12,* 104–115.

Sandelowski, M., & Barroso, J. (2002a). Finding the findings in qualitative studies. *Journal of Nursing Scholarship, 34,* 213–219.

Sandelowski, M., & Barroso, J. (2002b). Reading qualitative studies. *International Journal of Qualitative Methods, 1*(1), Article 5. Retrieved April 30, 2004, from http://www.ualberta.ca/~ijqm

Sandelowski, M., & Barroso, J. (2003a). Classifying the findings in qualitative studies. *Qualitative Health Research, 13,* 905–923.

Sandelowski, M., & Barroso, J. (2003b). Motherhood in the context of maternal HIV infection. *Research in Nursing & Health, 26,* 470–482.

Sandelowski, M., & Barroso, J. (2003c). Toward a metasynthesis of qualitative findings on motherhood in HIV-positive women. *Research in Nursing & Health, 26,* 153–170.

Sandelowski, M., Lambe, C., & Barroso, J. (2004). Stigma in HIV-positive women. *Journal of Nursing Scholarship, 36,* 122–128.

Sanjek, R. (Ed.). (1990). *Fieldnotes: The makings of anthropology.* Ithaca, NY: Cornell University Press.

Schatzman, L. (1991). Dimensional analysis: Notes on an alternative approach to the grounding of theory in qualitative research. In D. R. Maines (Ed.), *Social organization and social process: Essays in honor of Anselm Strauss* (pp. 303–314). New York: Aldine De Gruyter.

Scholes, J., Webb, C., Gray, M., Endacott, R., Miller, C., Jasper, M., et al. (2004). Making portfolios work in practice. *Journal of Advanced Nursing, 46,* 595–603.

Schwandt, T. A. (2000). Three epistemological stances for qualitative inquiry: Interpretivism, hermeneutics, and social constructionism. In N. K. Denzin & Y. S. Lincoln (Eds.), *Handbook of qualitative research* (2nd ed., pp. 189–213). Thousand Oaks, CA: Sage.

Schwartz-Barcott, D. (2003). Response to "concept advancement: Enhancing inductive validity." *Research and Theory for Nursing Practice: An International Journal, 17,* 169–174.

Schwartz-Barcott, D., & Kim, H. S. (2000). An expansion and elaboration of the Hybrid Model of Concept Development. In B. L. Rodgers & K. A. Knafl (Eds.), *Concept development in nursing: Foundations, techniques, and applications* (pp. 129–159). Philadelphia: W.B. Saunders.

Scott-Findlay, S., & Pollock, C. (2004). Evidence, research, knowledge: A call for conceptual clarity. *Worldviews on Evidence-Based Nursing, 1,* 92–97.

Semenic, S. E., Callister, L. C., & Feldman, P. (2004). Giving birth: The voices of orthodox Jewish women living in Canada. *JOGNN, 33,* 80–87.

Sharp, N. D., Pineros, S. L., Hsu, C., Starks, H., & Sales, A. E. (2004). A qualitative study to identify barriers and facilitators to implementation of pilot interventions in the Veterans Health Administration (VHA) Northwest Network. *Worldviews on Evidence-Based Nursing, 1,* 129–139.

Shearer, J. E. (2002). The concept of protection: A dimensional analysis and critique of a theory of protection. *Advances in Nursing Science, 25*(1), 65–78.

Shin, Y. H., Pender, N. J., & Yun, S. K. (2003). Using methodological triangulation for cultural verification of commitment to a plan for exercise scale among Korean adults with chronic diseases. *Research in Nursing & Health, 26*, 312–321.

Sidani, S., Epstein, D. R., & Moritz, P. (2003). An alternate paradigm for clinical nursing research: An exemplar. *Research in Nursing & Health, 26*, 244–255.

Siegel, S., & Castellan, N. J. (1988). *Nonparametric statistics for the behavioral sciences* (2nd ed.). New York: McGraw-Hill.

Silverman, D. (2000). Analyzing talk and text. In N. K. Denzin & Y. S. Lincoln (Eds.), *Handbook of qualitative research* (2nd ed., pp. 821–834). Thousand Oaks, CA: Sage.

Slakter, M. J., Wu, Y.-W., & Suzuki-Slakter, N. S. (1991). *, **, and ***: Statistical nonsense at the .00000 level. *Nursing Research, 40*, 248–249.

Sloane, P. D., Hoeffer, B., Mitchell, C. M., McKenzie, D. A., Barrisck, A. L., Rader, J., et al. (2004). Effect of person-centered showering and the towel bath on bathing-associated aggression, agitation, and discomfort in nursing home residents with dementia: A randomized, controlled trial. *Journal of the American Geriatrics Society, 52*, 1795–1804.

Smith, J., & McSherry, W. (2004). Spirituality and child development: A concept analysis. *Journal of Advanced Nursing, 45*, 307–315.

Smith, M. J., & Liehr, P. R. (Eds.). (2003). *Middle range theory for nursing*. New York: Springer.

Smith, R. A. P. (2004). Commentary. *Western Journal of Nursing Research, 26*, 167–169.

Smyth, K. A., & Yarandi, H. N. (1992). A path model of Type A and Type B responses to coping and stress in employed black women. *Nursing Research, 41*, 260–265.

Soriano, F. (1995). *Conducting needs assessments: A multidisciplinary approach*. Thousand Oaks, CA: Sage.

Spear, H. J. (2004). A follow-up case study on teenage pregnancy: "Havin' a baby isn't a nightmare, but it's really hard." *Pediatric Nursing, 30*, 120–125.

Stake, R. E. (2000). Case studies. In N. K. Denzin & Y. S. Lincoln (Eds.), *Handbook of qualitative research* (2nd ed., pp. 435–454). Thousand Oaks, CA: Sage.

Stephenson, W. (1953). *The study of behavior*. Chicago: University of Chicago Press.

Stevens, S. S. (1946). On the theory of scales of measurement. *Science, 103*, 677–680.

Strauss, A., & Corbin, J. (1990). *Basics of qualitative research: Grounded theory procedures and techniques*. Newbury Park, CA: Sage.

Strickland, O. L., Moloney, M. F., Dietrich, A. .S., Myerburg, J. D., Cotsonis, G. A., & Johnson, R. V. (2003). Measurement issues related to data collection on the World Wide Web. *Advances in Nursing Science, 26*(4), 246–256.

Stryer, D. B., Siegel, J. E., & Rodgers, A. B. (2004). Outcomes research: Priorities for an evolving field. *Medical Care, 42*(4 Suppl.), III-1–III-5.

Suppe, F. (Ed.). (1977). *The structure of scientific theories* (2nd ed.). Champaign, IL: University of Illinois Press.

Taft, L. B., Stolder, M. E., Knutson, A. B., Tamke, K., Platt, J., & Bowlds, T. (2004). Oral history: Validating contributions of elders. *Geriatric Nursing, 25*, 38–43.

Tang, S. T. (2003). Determinants of hospice home care use among terminally ill cancer patients. *Nursing Research, 52*, 217–225.

Tarnas, R. (1991). *The passion of the western mind: Understanding the ideas that have shaped our world view*. New York: Ballantine Books.

Taylor, C. (1979). Interpretation and the sciences of man. In P. Rabinow & W. M. Sullivan (Eds.), *Interpretive social science: A second look* (pp. 33–81). Berkeley: University of California Press.

Taylor, J. Y. (2004). Moving from surviving to thriving: African American women recovering from intimate male partner abuse. *Research and Theory for Nursing Practice: An International Journal, 18*, 35–50.

Taylor-Piliae, R. E., & Froelicher, E. S. (2004). The effectiveness of Tai Chi exercise in improving aerobic capacity: A meta-analysis. *Journal of Cardiovascular Nursing, 19*(1), 48–57.

Tedlock, B. (2000). Ethnography and ethnographic representation. In N. K. Denzin & Y. S. Lincoln (Eds.), *Handbook of qualitative research* (2nd ed., pp. 455–486). Thousand Oaks, CA: Sage.

Thomas, J. (1993). *Doing critical ethnography*. Newbury Park, CA: Sage.

References

Thomas, K. K. (2004). "Law unto themselves": Black women as patients and practitioners in North Carolina's campaign to reduce maternal and infant mortality, 1935–1953. *Nursing History Review, 12,* 47–66.

Thompson, J. L. (1990). Hermeneutic inquiry. In L. E. Moody (Ed.), *Advancing nursing science through research* (pp. 223–280, Volume 2). Newbury Park, CA: Sage.

Thompson, J. L. (2002). Dialogue. Which postmodernism? A critical response to 'Therapeutic touch and postmodernism in nursing.' *Nursing Philosophy, 3*(1), 58–62.

Thorndike, E. L. (1918). The nature, purposes and general methods of measurements of educational products. In E. L. Thorndike (Ed.), *The seventeenth yearbook of the National Society for the Study of Education* (Part 2). Bloomington, IL: Public School Publishing.

Thorne, S., Con, A., McGuinness, L., McPherson, G., & Harris, S. R. (2004). Health care communication issues in multiple sclerosis: An interpretive description. *Qualitative Health Research, 14,* 5–22.

Thorne, S. E., & Hayes, V. E. (Eds.). (1997). *Nursing praxis: Knowledge and action.* Thousand Oaks, CA: Sage.

Titler, M.G. (2004). Methods in translation science. *Worldviews on Evidence-Based Nursing, 1,* 38–48.

Tong, R. (1998). *Feminist thought: A more comprehensive introduction.* Boulder, CO: Westview Press.

Tourangeau, A. E., & McGilton, K. (2004). Measuring leadership practices of nurses using the leadership practices inventory. *Nursing Research, 53,* 182–189.

Tukey, J. W. (1977). *Exploratory data analysis.* Reading, MA: Addison-Wesley.

Tzeng, W-C., & Lipson, J. (2004). The cultural context of suicide stigma in Taiwan. *Qualitative Health Research, 14,* 345–358.

Ulrich, C. M., Soeken, K. L., & Miller, N. (2003). Ethical conflict associated with managed care. *Nursing Research, 52,* 168–175.

Uys, L. R. (2003). Aspects of the care of people with HIV/AIDS in South Africa. *Public Health Nursing, 20,* 271–280.

Van Maanen, J. (1988). *Tales of the field: On writing ethnography.* Chicago: University of Chicago Press.

van Manen, M. (1990). *Researching lived experience: Human Science for an active sensitive pedagogy.* London, Ontario, Canada: University of Western Ontario & State University of New York Press.

Varcoe, C. (2001). Abuse obscured: An ethnographic account of emergency nursing in relation to violence against women. *Canadian Journal of Nursing Research, 32*(4), 95–115.

Veeramah, V. (2004). Utilization of research findings by graduate nurses and midwives. *Journal of Advanced Nursing, 47,* 183–191.

Verran, J., & Ferketich, S. (1987a). Exploratory data analysis: Examining single distributions. *Western Journal of Nursing Research, 9,* 142–149.

Verran, J., & Ferketich, S. (1987b). Exploratory data analysis: Comparison of groups and variables. *Western Journal of Nursing Research, 9,* 617–625.

Villarruel, A. M., Harlow, S. D., Lopez, M., & Sowers, M. F. (2002). El cambio de vida: Conceptualizations of menopause and midlife among urban Latina women. *Research and Theory for Nursing Practice: An International Journal, 16,* 91–102.

Wagner, T. J. (1985). Smoking behavior of nurses in western New York. *Nursing Research, 34,* 58–60.

Wald, F. S., & Leonard, R. C. (1964). Towards development of nursing practice theory. *Nursing Research, 13,* 309–313.

Waldrop, M. M. (1992). *Complexity: The emerging science at the edge of order and chaos.* New York: Simon and Schuster.

Walker, L. O., & Avant, K. C. (1981/1988/1995/2005). *Strategies for theory construction in nursing* (1st–4th eds.). Norwalk, CT: Appleton & Lange.

Walker, L. O., & Montgomery, E. (1994). Maternal identity and role attainment: Long-term relations to children's development. *Nursing Research, 43,* 105–110.

Ward, S., Scarf Donovan, H., & Serlin, R. C. (2003). An alternative view on "An alternative paradigm." *Research in Nursing & Health, 26,* 256–259.

Ward-Griffin, C., Bol, N., Hay, K., & Dashnay, I. (2003). Relationships between families and registered nurses in long-term-care facilities: A critical analysis. *Canadian Journal of Nursing Research, 35*(4), 150–174.

Watson, J. (1985). *Nursing: Human science and human care. A theory of nursing.* Norwalk, CT: Appleton-Century-Crofts.

Watson, J. (1994). Poetizing as truth through language. In P. L. Chinn & J. Watson (Eds.), *Art and aesthetics in nursing* (pp. 3–17). New York: National League for Nursing Press.

Watson, J. (1995). Postmodernism and knowledge development in nursing. *Nursing Science Quarterly, 8,* 60–64.

Watson, J. (1999). *Postmodern nursing and beyond.* Edinburgh, Scotland: Churchill Livingstone.

Watson, N. M., Brink, C. A., Zimmer, J. G., & Mayer, R. D. (2003). Use of the Agency for Health Care Policy and Research Urinary Incontinence Guideline in nursing homes. *Journal of the American Geriatrics Society, 51,* 1779–1786.

Webb, E. J., Campbell, D. T., Schwartz, R. B., Sechrest, L., & Grove, J. B. (1981). *Nonreactive measures in the social sciences* (2nd ed.). Boston: Houghton Mifflin.

Weiss, S. J. (1995). Contemporary empiricism. In A. Omery, C. E. Kasper, & G. G. Page (Eds.), *In search of nursing science* (pp. 13–26). Thousand Oaks, CA: Sage.

Weitzman, E. A. (2000). Software and qualitative research. In N. K. Denzin & Y. S. Lincoln (Eds.), *Handbook of qualitative research* (2nd ed., pp. 803–820). Thousand Oaks, CA: Sage.

Wewers, M. E., & Lowe, N. K. (1990). A critical review of visual analogue scales in the measurement of clinical phenomena. *Research in Nursing & Health, 13,* 227–236.

Whitney, J. D., Stotts, N. A., Goodson, W. H., & Janson-Bjerklie, S. (1993). The effects of activity and bed rest on tissue oxygen tension, perfusion, and plasma volume. *Nursing Research, 42,* 349–355.

Whittemore, R., Chase, S. K., & Mandle, C. L. (2001). Validity in qualitative research. *Qualitative Health Research, 11,* 522–537.

Wikoff, R. L., & Miller, P. (1991). Canonical analysis in nursing research. *Nursing Research, 40,* 367–370.

Wilde, M. H. (2002). Urine flowing: A phenomenological study of living with a urinary catheter. *Research in Nursing and Health, 25,* 14–24.

Williams, M. A., Oberst, M. T., & Bjorklund, B. (1994). Early outcomes after hip fracture among women discharged home and to nursing homes. *Research in Nursing & Health, 17,* 175–183.

Williamson, G. R., Webb, C., & Abelson-Mitchell, N. (2004). Developing lecturer practitioner roles using action research. *Journal of Advanced Nursing, 47,* 153–164.

Wilson, J. (1963/1970). *Thinking with concepts.* New York: Cambridge University Press.

Wooldridge, P. J., Schmitt, M. H., Skipper, J. K., & Leonard, R. C. (1983). *Behavioral science & nursing theory.* St. Louis, MO: C.V. Mosby.

Workman, M. L., & Livingston, G. K. (1993). Testing the sensitivity of a biologic assay for mutagenicity. *Nursing Research, 42,* 373–375.

Wu, Y-W. B. (1995). Hierarchical linear models: A multilevel data analysis technique. *Nursing Research, 44,* 123–126.

Wuest, J. (1995). Feminist grounded theory: An exploration of the congruency and tensions between two traditions in knowledge discovery. *Qualitative Health Research, 5,* 125–137.

Wuest, J. (1998). Setting boundaries: A strategy for precarious ordering of women's caring demands. *Research in Nursing & Health, 21,* 39–49.

Wuest, J., & Merritt-Gray, M. (2001). Beyond survival: Reclaiming self after leaving an abusive male partner. *Canadian Journal of Nursing Research, 32*(4), 79–94.

Yarcheski, A., Mahon, N. E., Yarcheski, T. J., & Cannella, B. L. (2004). A meta-analysis of predictors of positive health practices. *Journal of Nursing Scholarship, 36,* 102–108.

Yen, M., & Lo, L-H. (2002). Examining test-retest reliability: An intra-class correlation approach. *Nursing Research, 51,* 59–62.

Yin, R. K. (2003). *Case study research: Design and methods* (3rd ed.). Thousand Oaks, CA: Sage.

Yura, H., & Torres, G. (1975). *Today's conceptual frameworks with the baccalaureate nursing programs* (NLN Pub. No. 15-1558, pp. 17–75). New York: National League for Nursing.

Zachariah, R. (1994). Maternal-fetal attachment: Influence of mother-daughter and husband-wife relationships. *Research in Nursing & Health, 17,* 37–44.

Zauszniewski, J. A., & Suresky, J. (2003, December 19). Evidence for psychiatric nursing practice: An analysis of three years of published research. *Online Journal of Issues in Nursing.* Retrieved July 12, 2004, from http://nursingworld.org/ojin/hirsh/topic4/tpc4 1.htm

Zeller, R., Good, M., Anderson, G. C., & Zeller, D. (1997). Strengthening experimental design by balancing confounding variables across eight treatment groups. *Nursing Research, 46,* 345–349.

References

Zerwic, J. J., Ryan, C. J., DeVon, H. A., & Drell, M. J. (2003). Treatment seeking for acute my-ocardial infarction symptoms: Differences in delay across sex and race. *Nursing Research, 52,* 159–167.

Zimmer, J. G., Watson, N., & Treat, A. (1984). Behavioral problems among patients in skilled nursing facilities. *American Journal of Public Health, 74,* 1118–1121.

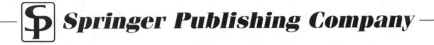

Springer Publishing Company

Encyclopedia of Nursing Research

Second Edition

Joyce J. Fitzpatrick, PhD, RN, FAAN, Editor

Meredith Wallace, PhD, RN, CS-ANP, Associate Editor

The push toward evidence-based practice makes it crucial for all nurses to be familiar with basic research terminology, methods, databases, and seminal research in specific clinical areas. This comprehensive reference is a "one-stop" resource for everything you need to know about nursing research and its utilization. Compiled by the world's leading authorities in nursing research, this thoroughly updated new edition presents key terms and concepts by over 200 contributors, with nearly 30% newly added terms. It is written for nurse researchers, graduate students, and clinicians. Extensive cross references assist in the information-seeking process.

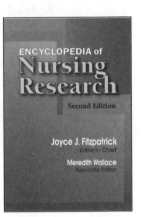

Partial Contents:

- Advanced Practice Nursing
- Applied Research
- Clinical Nursing Research
- Computer-Based Documentation
- Concept Analysis
- Data Management
- Discourse Analysis
- Ethics of Research
- Family Caregiving to Frail Elderly
- Feminist Research Methodology
- Geriatrics
- Henderson's Model
- Internet
- Journals in Nursing Research

- Measurement and Scales
- Nursing Informatics
- Nursing Theoretical Models
- Outcomes Measures
- Populations and Aggregates
- Qualitative and Quantitative Research
- Research Utilization
- Statistical Techniques
- Telehealth
- Unified Language Systems
- Validity
- World Wide Web

2005   837pp   0-8261-9812-0   hardcover

11 West 42nd Street, New York, NY 10036-8002 • Fax: 212-941-7842
Order Toll-Free: 877-687-7476 • Order On-line: www.springerpub.com

SP *Springer Publishing Company*

Research in Nursing and Health
Second Edition
Understanding and Using Quantitative and Qualitative Methods

Carol Noll Hoskins, PhD, RN, FAAN
Carla Mariano, EdD, RN, HNC, FAAIM
with contributors

This updated edition offers the reader a step-by-step guide to conducting research and to understanding the research studies done by others. It describes both quantitative and qualitative investigations. The book is written in outline format, for quick reference. An important feature of the new edition is an extensive listing of online databases and knowledge resources. Graduate students and nurse researchers will find this an easily accessible source of valuable information.

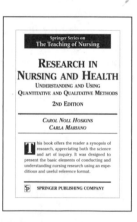

Partial Contents:

- Introduction to Research, *C. Hoskins & C. Mariano*
- The Research Question, *C. Hoskins & C. Mariano*
- A Review of the Literature Using Online & Print Sources, *B. Carty et al.*
- Research Designs, *C. Hoskins & C. Mariano*
- Sampling Methods: Basic Issues and Concepts, *C. Mariano & J. Giacquinta*
- Principles of Measurement, *C. Hoskins & H. Feldman*
- Data Analysis and Interpretation, *C. Hoskins & C. Mariano*
- Product of the Inquiry: The Research Report, *C. Hoskins & C. Mariano*
- Guide to Critique of Quantitative Research—with Examples and Practice Studies, *C. Hoskins*
- Appendices: Suggested Guide for Abstracting Research Studies; Guide to Critique of Philosophical Research; Issues of Control and Validity: Quantitative Studies; Testing Hypotheses with an Exemplar Study: Statistical Significance, Error, Directionality, and Power

2004 200pp 0-8261-1616-7 softcover

11 West 42nd Street, New York, NY 10036-8002 • Fax: 212-941-7842
Order Toll-Free: 877-687-7476 • Order On-line: www.springerpub.com